Series editor
Daniel Horton-Szar
BSc (Hons) MBBS (Hons)
GP Registrar
Northgate Medical Practice
Canterbury

Faculty advisor
Dr Kevin Harris
Department of Medicine and
  Therapeutics
University of Leicester School of
  Medicine
Leicester General Hospital
Gwendolen Road
Leicester

Renal and Urinary System

SECOND EDITION

Shreelata Datta

BSc (Hons)
Imperial College School of Medicine
Princes Road
South Kensington
London

First edition authors
Nisha Mirpuri, Pratiksha Patel

M Mosby

Edinburgh • London • New York • Oxford • Philadelphia • St Louis • Sydney • Toronto 2002

MOSBY
An imprint of Elsevier Science Limited

Commissioning editor	**Alex Stibbe**
Project Manager	**Frances Affleck**
Project Development Manager	**Duncan Fraser**
Designer	**Andy Chapman**
Cover Design	**Kevin Faerber**
Illustration Manager	**Mick Ruddy**

First edition © 1998, Mosby International Ltd
This edition © 2003, Elsevier Science Ltd. All rights reserved

First edition 1998
Second edition 2003
  Reprinted 2003

ISBN 07234 32503

British Library Cataloguing in Publication Data
A catalogue record for this book is available from the British Library

Library of Congress Cataloging in Publication Data
A catalog record for this book is available from the Library of Congress

Note
Medical knowledge is constantly changing. Standard safety precautions must be followed, but as new research and clinical experience broaden our knowledge, changes in treatment and drug therapy may become necessary or appropriate. Readers are advised to check the most current product information provided by the manufacturer of each drug to be administered to verify the recommended dose, the method and duration of administration, and contraindications. It is the responsibility of the practitioner, relying on experience and knowledge of the patient, to determine dosages and the best treatment for each individual patient. Neither the Publisher nor the authors and editors assume any liability for any injury and/or damage to persons or property arising from this publication.
The Publisher

Typeset by SNP Best-set Typesetter Ltd., Hong Kong
Printed in Spain

The publisher's policy is to use paper manufactured from sustainable forests

ELSEVIER SCIENCE
your source for books,
journals and multimedia
in the health sciences
www.elsevierhealth.com

The
publisher's
policy is to use
paper manufactured
from sustainable forests

Preface

The words 'glomerulonephritis' and 'detrusor instability' are enough to strike fear into the hearts of the bravest of medical students, with the renal and urinary systems remaining a challenge for undergraduate students to come to terms with. It is often viewed as a specialist area, although it is affected by many of the common systemic diseases.

Crash Course: Renal and Urinary Systems aims to present essential information in an accessible and student-friendly manner. It has been structured to combine the scientific core with the relevant clinical detail, and thus fits in with integrated medical course. Wherever possible, the text has been supported with diagrams, images, algorithms and tables to simplify and summarize complex principles. In addition, students have the opportunity to test their knowledge using the self-assessment sections throughout the book.

I hope you find this book useful as an overview to guide you through the complexities of the renal and urinary systems—from the tip of the urethra to the heart of the glomerulus!

Shreelata Datta

Diseases of the urinary tract have traditionally been seen as a challenge for medical students. To address this *Crash Course: Renal and Urinary Systems* is written in a way that allows students to develop their knowledge in a balanced and logical way while stimulating them to continue with self-directed learning.

As with all *Crash Course* books, the text is written by a medical student with expert input from a Faculty Advisor—me—and the Series Editor. This approach has ensured that the book will provide students with a solid, accurate, user-friendly and relevant overview of the subject. The integrated approach between basic and clinical sciences provides the appropriate theoretical basis for solving the kind of problems that are commonly encountered in clinical practice.

This second edition has been extensively revised, building, where appropriate, on the first edition using readers' feedback and suggestions. The text has been updated yet retains its concise and clear style. New images of disease have been added to the already plentiful illustrations and the Self-assessment section contains new MCQs, SAQs and essay topics.

It's hoped that this book provides students with a useful supplement to their lecture notes and a concise and comprehensive revision aid for testing their knowledge of this fascinating subject.

Dr Kevin Harris
Faculty Advisor

In the six years since the first editions were published, there have been many changes in medicine, and in the way it is taught. These second editions have been largely rewritten to take these changes into account, and keep *Crash Course* up to date for the twenty-first century. New material has been added to include recent research and all pharmacological and disease management information has been updated in line with current best practice. We've listened to feedback from hundreds of students who have been using *Crash Course* and have improved the structure and layout of the books accordingly: pathology material has been closely integrated with the relevant basic medical science; there are more MCQs and the clarity of text and figures is better than ever.

The principles on which we developed the series remain the same, however. Medicine is a huge subject, and the last thing a student needs when exams are looming is to waste time assembling information from different sources, and wading through pages of irrelevant detail. As before, *Crash Course* brings you all the information you need, in compact, manageable volumes that integrate basic medical science with clinical practice. We still tread the fine line between producing clear, concise text and providing enough detail for those aiming at distinction. The series is still written by medical students with recent exam experience, and checked for accuracy by senior faculty members from across the UK.

I wish you the best of luck in your future careers!

Dr Dan Horton-Szar
Series Editor

Acknowledgements

I would like to thank Dr Harris and Dr Dan Horton-Szar, who helped prevent many a sleepless night, and all the team at Elsevier.

Thanks also go to my family and friends, who have tirelessly put up with my moans and groans and supported me over the past year.

Figure acknowledgements

Figs 1.9, 1.10, 3.14 and 3.19 redrawn with kind permission from C J Lote. Principles of Renal Physiology, 4th edition. Kluwer Academic Publishers, 2000

Figs 2.7 and 2.27 adapted with permission from A Stevens and J Lowe. Human Histology, 2nd edition. Mosby, 1997

Fig 4.1 adapted with permission from C Page, M Curtis, M Sutter, M Walker and B Hoffman. Integrated Pharmacology. Mosby, 1997

Fig 8.12A reproduced with permission from G Williams and N P Mallick. Color Atlas of Renal Diseases. Mosby 1994

Fig 8.20 redrawn with permission from L Impey. Obstetrics and Gynaecology. Blackwell Science, 1999

Dedication

To my parents, who made me who I am today, and to my Science teachers who first inspired me.

Contents

BASIC MEDICAL SCIENCE OF THE RENAL AND URINARY SYSTEMS

1. Basic Principles

Overview of the kidney and urinary tract

Structural organization of the kidney and urinary tract

The kidneys lie in the retroperitoneum on the posterior abdominal wall on either side of the vertebral column (T11–L3). The right kidney is displaced by the liver, so is 12mm lower than the left kidney. The adult kidney is approximately 11cm long and 6cm wide, with a mass of 140g. Each kidney is composed of two main regions:

- An outer dark brown cortex.
- An inner pale medulla and renal pelvis.

The renal pelvis contains the major renal blood vessels and the origins of the ureter. Each kidney consists of 1 million nephrons, which span the cortex and medulla and are bound together by connective tissue containing blood vessels, nerves and lymphatics.

The kidneys form the upper part of the urinary tract. The urine produced by the kidneys is transported to the bladder by two ureters. The lower urinary tract consists of the bladder and the urethra.

Approximately 1–1.5L urine are produced by the kidneys each day—the volume and osmolality vary according to fluid intake and fluid loss.

The urinary tract epithelium is impermeable to water and solutes, unlike the nephrons in the kidney, so the composition of the urine is not altered as it is transported to the bladder. The bladder contents are emptied via the urethra, expulsion from the body being controlled by an external sphincter. Both the upper and lower urinary tract are innervated by the autonomic nervous system.

Figure 1.1 shows the anatomy of the kidneys and urinary tract.

Functions of the kidney and the urinary tract

1. **Excretion:** of waste products and drugs—this involves selective reabsorption and excretion of substances as they pass through the nephron.
2. **Regulation:** of body fluid volume and ionic composition. The kidneys have a major role in homeostasis (the maintenance of a constant internal environment) and are also involved in maintaining the acid–base balance.
3. **Endocrine:** the kidneys are involved in the synthesis of renin (which generates angiotensin I from angiotensinogen, and thus has a role in blood pressure and sodium balance), erythropoietin (which controls erythrocyte production) and prostaglandins (involved in vasodilation).
4. **Metabolism:** of vitamin D and low-molecular-weight proteins. The kidney is a major site for the catabolism of several hormones, such as insulin, parathyroid hormone and calcitonin.

Fluid compartments of the body

Body fluids

Body fluids are divided into:
- Intracellular fluid (ICF), the fluid within cells.
- Extracellular fluid (ECF).

ECF is divided into:
- Plasma—ECF within the vascular system, i.e. the non-cellular component of blood.
- Interstitial fluid (ISF)—ECF outside the vascular system (and separated from plasma by the capillary endothelium).
- Transcellular fluid (TCF)—ECF (e.g. synovial fluid, aqueous and vitreous humour, cerebrospinal fluid) separated from plasma by the capillary endothelium and an additional epithelial layer that has specialized functions (Fig. 1.2).

Water is a major component of the human body. Approximately 63% of an adult male and 52% of an adult female is water (i.e. 45L in a 70kg male, 36L in a 70kg female). This difference is due to the fact that

3

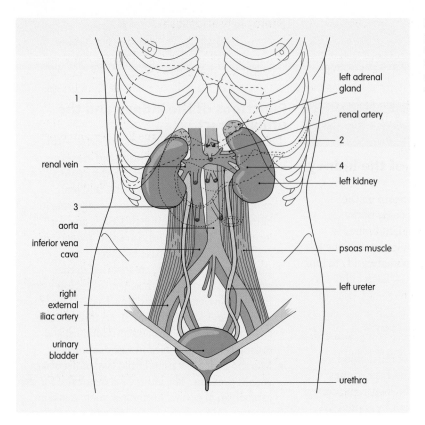

Fig. 1.1 Anatomy of the posterior abdominal wall showing the renal and urinary system. 1, Liver; 2, stomach; 3, second part of the duodenum; 4, pancreas.

left adrenal gland

renal artery

2

4

left kidney

renal vein

1

3

aorta

inferior vena cava

right external iliac artery

urinary bladder

psoas muscle

left ureter

urethra

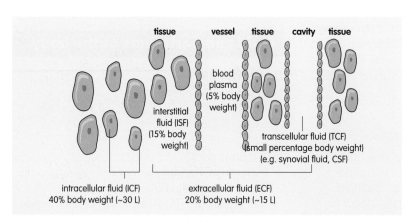

tissue   vessel   tissue   cavity   tissue

blood plasma (5% body weight)

interstitial fluid (ISF) (15% body weight)

transcellular fluid (TCF) (small percentage body weight) (e.g. synovial fluid, CSF)

intracellular fluid (ICF) 40% body weight (~30 L)

extracellular fluid (ECF) 20% body weight (~15 L)

Fig. 1.2 Fluid compartments of the body.

females have a higher proportion of body fat, which has a low water content. One-third of total body water (TBW) is ECF (about 15 L in a 70 kg male) and two-thirds is ICF (about 30 L in a 70 kg male).

Osmolarity and osmolality
Basic concepts
Osmosis is the net passage of a solvent through a semi-permeable membrane from a less concentrated solution to a more concentrated solution. This occurs until both solutions reach the same concentration (equilibrium). The osmotic effect can be measured as an osmotic pressure. This is the pressure at which water is drawn into a solution across a semi-permeable membrane. Thus, the more concentrated the solution (i.e. the higher the solute content), the greater the osmotic pressure. Hydrostatic pressure is the pressure needed to be applied to the region

containing the solute to prevent the net entry of water.

Osmolarity is the total solute concentration of a solution—the number of osmotically active particles in solution. The higher the osmolarity, the lower the water concentration. 1 Osmole (Osmol) = 1 mole of solute particles.

Osmolarity versus osmolality

Osmolarity measures the molar concentration of solute particles per litre of solution (mOsmol/L). *Osmolality* is the molar concentration of solute particles per kilogram of solvent (water) (mOsmol/kgH$_2$O). Figure 1.3 illustrates the differences between osmolality and osmolarity.

- Normal body fluid osmolality is between 285 and 295 mOsmol/kgH$_2$O.
- Urine osmolality may vary between 60 and 1400 mOsmol/kgH$_2$O.

Plasma osmolality can be calculated from sodium ion (Na$^+$), potassium ion (K$^+$), urea, and glucose concentrations using the formula:

Plasma osmolality = 2(Na$^+$ + K$^+$) + urea + glucose

Isotonicity and isosmoticity

Changes in the extracellular osmolarity can cause cells to shrink or swell because water will move across the plasma membrane by osmosis into or out of the cells to maintain equilibrium. Therefore, an important function of the kidneys is to regulate the excretion of water in the urine so that the osmolarity of the ECF remains nearly constant despite wide variations in intake or extrarenal losses of salt and water. This prevents damage to the cells from excess swelling and shrinkage:

- If cells are placed in a solution over 295 mOsmol (hypertonic solution), they shrink as water moves out into the solution.
- If cells are placed in a solution of 285–295 mOsmol/kgH$_2$O (isotonic solution, i.e. 0.9% saline), there is no net movement of water by osmosis and no swelling or shrinkage. This is because an isotonic solution has the same osmolarity as normal body fluid.
- If cells are placed in a solution less than 285 mOsmol (hypotonic solution), they swell as water enters from the solution.

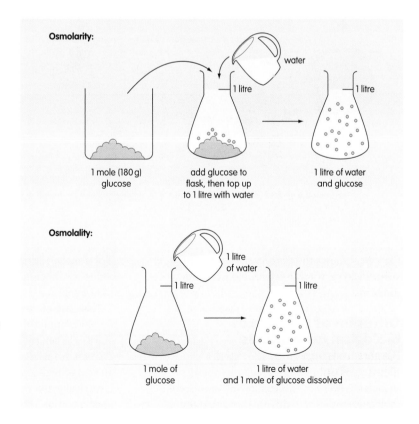

Fig. 1.3 Osmolarity can be described as 1 mole of glucose added to water, dissolved to make up to 1 litre. Osmolality is the addition of 1 litre of water to one mole of glucose (adapted from Lote CJ 2000 Principles of renal physiology, 4th edn. Kluwer Academic Publishers, p 4–5).

- **Isosmoticity:** this refers to solutions with the same solution concentration per kilogram water (e.g. 0.9% saline and 5% dextrose).
- **Isotonicity:** this refers to solutions that do not cause any change in cell volume (e.g. 285–295 mOsmol/L of non-permeable solute).

Thus, different isotonic solutions are isosmotic, but solutions that are isosmotic to plasma are not necessarily isotonic.

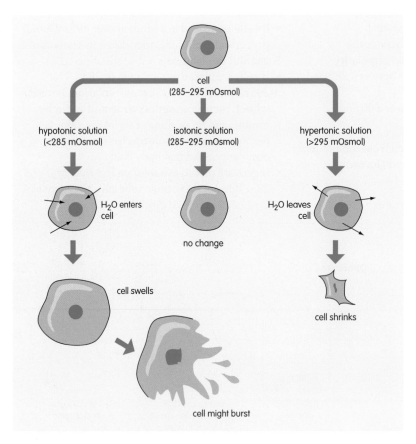

Fig. 1.4 Cell changes induced by hypotonic, isotonic and hypertonic solutions.

Figure 1.4 shows the changes in the cells brought about by hypertonic, isotonic and hypotonic solutions.

Diffusion of ions across biological membranes
Passive transport

Biological membranes (e.g. cell membranes) are selectively permeable, allowing only small molecules and ions to diffuse through them.

The concentration gradient and electrical gradient influence the movement of these molecules into or out of cells.

The rate of diffusion of different molecules depends upon their shape, size, weight and electrical charge. When solutions either side of a membrane contain diffusible ions only, ions move passively from an area of high ionic concentration down the electrical gradient to an area of lower ionic concentration. This occurs until equilibrium is reached, when the ion distribution on either side of the membrane will be as follows:

Side A (diffusible cations × diffusible anions)
    = Side B (diffusible cations × diffusible anions)

The Gibbs–Donnan effect
Proteins are negatively charged molecules that are so large that they cannot diffuse across membranes. Thus, if proteins are present on one side of the membrane (side A), they act as anions and attract positive ions (cations) from side B. Cations diffuse across the membrane to the more negative side A, and thus maintain electrical neutrality. As a result, side A will not only contain non-diffusible proteins, but also the cations from side B—and therefore will have a greater number of total ions. Consequently, the osmotic pressure on side A will be greater. This encourages the entry of water, unless the osmotic pressure difference is counterbalanced by hydrostatic pressure on side B (Fig. 1.5).

Cell membranes are permeable to:
- Potassium ions (K^+).
- Chloride ions (Cl^-).
- Sodium ions (Na^+).

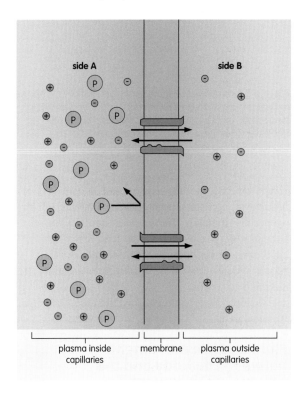

$\underbrace{\text{plasma inside capillaries}} \quad \underbrace{\text{membrane}} \quad \underbrace{\text{plasma outside capillaries}}$

side A   side B

Fig. 1.5 The Gibbs–Donnan effect. $\oplus$, diffusible cation; $\ominus$ diffusible anion; P, impermeable molecule (e.g. protein).

Active transport
Na^+ permeability is 1/50th K^+ permeability. The primary active transport mechanism uses energy in the form of adenosine triphosphate (ATP) to actively pump Na^+ out of and K^+ into the cells against a concentration gradient. This sodium pump is composed of several proteins and lies within the cell membrane of all cells. Cl^- ions diffuse passively out of the cell across the cell membrane because there is an overall negative charge within the cell. This leads to a higher concentration of Cl^- ions outside the cells. At equilibrium, the cell has a net negative charge ($-70mV$).

According to the Gibbs–Donnan effect, there should be more ions inside the cell than outside because of the effects of anionic proteins. This is balanced in biological systems by the sodium pump as Na^+ is effectively non-diffusible.

Solute transport can be
- Passive—i.e. spontaneous, down an electrochemical gradient. This requires no energy.
- Active—i.e. against an electrochemical gradient. This is energy dependent.

Fluid movement between body compartments
At any one moment, body fluid compartments have a relatively constant yet dynamic composition. Equilibrium is maintained by the continual transfer of fluid between the different compartments.

Exchange between ECF and ICF
Water diffuses freely across cell membranes so that equilibrium is reached between the ICF and ECF. Any change in the ionic concentration of the ICF or ECF is followed by the movement of water between these compartments.
- Na^+ is the most important extracellular osmotically active ion.
- K^+ is the most important intracellular osmotically active ion.

Exchange between plasma and ISF

The capillary endothelium separates plasma (within the circulatory system) from interstitial fluid (ISF—outside the circulatory system). Water and ions move between these two compartments— 90% of ions by simple diffusion and 10% by filtration.

Ion filtration between plasma and ISF relies on:

- The arterial end of the capillary, which has a hydrostatic pressure of 32mmHg, forcing fluid out of the capillary plasma into the ISF.
- Proteins that are too large to cross the capillary endothelial cells, and therefore remain in the plasma, creating a colloid osmotic (or oncotic) pressure (25mmHg).
- The venous end of the capillary having an osmotic pressure of 25mmHg. This is greater than the hydrostatic pressure (12mmHg), causing fluid to move out of the ISF and re-enter the capillary plasma.

The movement of fluid across a capillary wall between the plasma and ISF is illustrated in Fig.1.6.

Hydrostatic pressure depends upon:

- Arteriole blood pressure.
- Arteriole resistance (which determines the extent to which blood pressure is transferred to the capillary).
- Venous blood pressure.

Osmotic pressure (25mmHg) is produced by plasma proteins (17mmHg—oncotic pressure) and the imbalance of ions—there are more ions (e.g. Na^+) within the capillary than outside. This is due to the presence of negatively charged proteins and the Gibbs–Donnan effect.

Water diffusion is controlled by two forces:
- Hydrostatic pressure (within the vascular system only).
- Osmotic pressure (from plasma proteins).

Exchange between interstitial fluid and lymphatic vessels

Plasma proteins and fluid lost from the vascular system are filtered into the ISF, and taken up by the

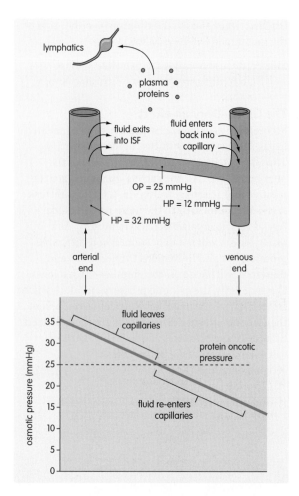

Fig. 1.6 Starling forces—factors involved in fluid exchange between the plasma and ISF across a capillary wall. HP, hydrostatic pressure; OP, oncotic pressure. *Note*: HP decreases from the arterial to the venous end of the capillary; OP is constant throughout.

lymphatic system. This is composed of a network of lymphatic capillaries in all organs and tissues, which eventually drain into the venous system via the thoracic duct in the neck. These lymphatic capillaries are very permeable to protein and thus return both the fluid and plasma proteins to the circulatory system.

The ionic composition of the fluid compartments is shown in Fig. 1.7.

Fluid and ion movement between the body and the external environment

There is a continuous exchange of body fluids with the external environment, but there must be a

Composition of fluid compartments			
Component	Plasma	ECF	ICF*
Na$^+$ (mmol/L)	142	145	12
K$^+$ (mmol/L)	4	4.1	150
Cl$^-$ (mmol/L)	103	113	4
HCO$_3^-$ (mmol/L)	25	27	12
proteins (g/L)	60	0	25
osmolality (mOsm/kg H$_2$O)	280	280	280
compartment volume (L)	3.0	12.0	30

*ICF compartment is not the same throughout the body; it varies with different types of cells

Fig. 1.7 Composition of the body fluid compartments.

Water intake and output			
Water intake (mL)		Water output (mL)	
drink	1500	lungs	400
food	500	skin	400
metabolism	400	faeces	100
		urine	1500
total	2400	total	2400

Fig. 1.8 Distribution of daily water ingestion and losses.

balance between intake and output, as body weight is consistent from day to day.

Daily water intake and output are shown in Fig. 1.8. Water lost from the lungs varies with the climate (e.g. in very dry climates over 400ml per day is lost). Insensible losses are those due to evaporation of water from the skin (i.e. not sweat). Sweating ('sensible perspiration') is an additional loss, which acts as a homeostatic mechanism to maintain constant body temperature. Urinary loss can be adjusted according to the needs of the body, and water intake. The amount of water lost in defecation can also vary, and is increased greatly in diarrhoea.

Daily water intake can fluctuate considerably and can be altered according to need (i.e. thirst mechanism). Water derived from metabolism is the result of oxidation of food. Despite these variations, the body's ionic concentration is maintained within the normal range by the kidney's homeostatic mechanisms, which include control of tubular reabsorption of filtered Na$^+$—and to a lesser extent K$^+$—as well as regulating water reabsorption.

Whereas water intake can be controlled, normally, the minimum water loss from urine, lungs, skin and faeces cannot fall below 1200mL/day. Thus, if there is no water intake, dehydration occurs, eventually resulting in death within a few days.

Measuring body fluid compartments
Dilution principle
The dilution principle is used to measure fluid volume if fluids cannot be directly measured or extracted from the container or compartment holding them. This allows measuring in situ. A substance that will mix completely and uniformly in the fluid compartment is used to allow all of the volume present to be measured, e.g. a dye. Allowances must be made for the excretion and metabolism of the selected indicator by the body.

$$V_D = \frac{Q_A - Q_H}{C}$$

Where V_D = volume of distribution; Q_A = quantity administered; Q_H = quantity metabolized after 10h; C = concentration.

Two methods are used:
- Single injection method.
- Constant infusion method.

Single injection method
This is used for test substances with a slow rate of excretion from the compartment being measured, and is carried out as follows:
1. A known amount of test substance is injected intravenously.
2. Plasma concentration is determined at intervals.
3. A graph (log concentration against time scale) is plotted (Fig. 1.9).
4. The straight portion back to the start (i.e. time 0) is extrapolated—this gives the concentration of substance assuming it had distributed evenly and instantly.

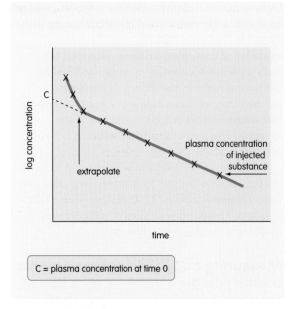

Fig. 1.9 The dilution principle: single injection method, showing the plasma concentration of an injected substance.

Fig. 1.10 The dilution principle: constant infusion method, showing the plasma concentration of an infused substance.

Using this method:

Compartment volume =
$$\frac{\text{Amount injected}}{\text{Concentration at zero time}}$$

Constant infusion method
This is used for test substances that are excreted rapidly and is carried out as follows:
1. A loading dose of the test substance is injected intravenously.
2. The test substance is infused at a rate to match the excretion rate.
3. Plasma concentration is measured at intervals.
4. When the substance comes to equilibrium, the plasma concentration is constant (Fig. 1.10).
5. The infusion is stopped and urine collected until all the test substance has been excreted.

Using this method:

Amount excreted = Amount present in the body at the time the infusion was stopped

and:

Compartment volume (L) =
$$\frac{\text{Amount excreted (mg)}}{\text{Plasma concentration (mg/L)}}$$

Measurement of plasma volume, red cell volume and blood volume
Plasma volume, blood volume and red cell volume are measured as follows:
- **Plasma volume:** this is measured using the dilution principle. The test substance needs to remain within the vascular system (e.g. high-molecular-weight substance). Radio-iodinated human serum albumin or Evans Blue dye are commonly used.
  Normal plasma volume = 3 L.
- **Blood volume:** derived from the kidney plasma volume and the haematocrit (% of red blood cells in total blood volume). For example, if the haematocrit is 45%, the plasma volume is 55% of blood volume (measure plasma volume as above and blood volume = plasma volume × 100/55).
  Normal blood volume = 5 L.

- **Red cell volume:** this can be derived from plasma volume and haematocrit or measured by direct dilution, using radiolabelled red blood cells.

Measurement of extracellular fluid (ECF)

As ECF is made up of several compartments (plasma, interstitial fluid and transcellular fluid), it is difficult to measure accurately. A substance that will diffuse quickly across the endothelial barriers into the ISF, but not into the cells, is required. Substances used include:

- Insulin (can be excluded from bone and cartilage).
- Mannitol.
- Thiosulphate (most commonly used).
- Radiosulfate.
- Thiocyanate.
- Radiochloride or radiosodium (these substances cannot be completely excluded from cells).

A known amount of the selected indicator is injected intravenously and the ECF volume is calculated using the dilution principle. It is difficult to measure the transcellular fluid (TCF) because it is separated from the capillaries by another membrane in addition to the capillary membrane.
Normal ECF volume = 15 L.

Measurement of interstitial fluid (ISF)

This cannot be measured directly and is calculated using the following equation:

ISF (12 L) = ECF (15 L) – plasma volume (3 L)

Measurement of total body water

Isotopes of water are used as markers (deuterium oxide or tritiated water) to measure total body water (TBW). A normal value in a 70-kg man is 63% (i.e. 45 L) and in a 70-kg woman, 52% (36 L), being lower in women because of their greater proportion of body fat.

Measurement of transcellular fluid (TCF)

As this compartment is separated from the rest of the ECF by a membrane, the substances used to measure the ECF do not cross into this compartment. Thus TCF is included in the TBW, but excluded from the ECF:

TBW = ECF + ICF + TCF

There is a large turnover—about 20 L/day in the gastrointestinal tract.

Figure 1.11 summarizes the methods used to measure the different fluid volumes.

Summary of fluid volume measurements in a 70 kg individual		
Fluid volume	**Normal volume**	**Method of measurement**
plasma volume	3 L	radio-iodinated human serum albumin or Evans blue dye
blood volume	5 L	determined from the haematocrit
red cell volume	2 L	• measured from plasma volume and haematocrit • direct dilution
extracellular fluid (ECF)	15 L	indirect measurement using an injected substance (e.g. inulin)
intracellular fluid (ICF)	28 L	ICF = TBW - ECF - TCF
interstitial fluid (ISF)	12 L	calculated from ECF and plasma volume
total body water (TBW)	63% of total mass (men) 53% of total mass (women)	isotopes of water are used as markers
transcellular fluid (TCF)	20 L/day turnover in the gut	TCF = TBW - ECF - ICF

Fig. 1.11 Summary of of fluid compartments and their measurement in an individual weighing 70kg.

- Describe the location and composition of the kidneys.
- Summarize the main functions of the kidney.
- Name the different fluid compartments within the body, stating their relative proportions and values.
- Distinguish between osmolarity and osmolality, defining the units of measurement for each.
- Explain how the following influence the distribution of ions across a semi-permeable membrane:
  (a) Concentration gradient.
  (b) Electrical gradient.
  (c) Proteins.
- What is the role of the lymphatic system in fluid movement?
- Describe the routes by which water and ions enter and leave the body, giving the relevant values.
- Outline the difference between the two methods used in the dilution principle.
- Discuss why it is important to use high-molecular-weight plasma proteins when measuring plasma volume.
- Explain why interstitial fluid must be measured indirectly.

2. Organization of the Kidneys

Development of the kidneys

The kidneys pass through three developmental stages (Fig. 2.1):

- **Pronephros:** the most primitive system, developing in the cervical region of the embryo during the fourth week of gestation. It is non-functional and regresses soon after its formation, leaving behind a nephritic duct.
- **Mesonephros:** develops in the lumbar region and functions for a short period. It consists of excretory tubules with their own collecting ducts known as mesonephric ducts. These drain into the nephritic ducts.
- **Metanephros:** develops in the sacral region at approximately 5 weeks gestation and eventually forms the final adult kidneys. It becomes functional in the latter half of the pregnancy.

The functional unit of the kidney—the nephron—develops from the fusion of the:

- **Metanephric blastema**, which is from the nephrogenic cord (part of the intermediate mesoderm). This forms the nephron tubular system from the glomerulus to the distal tubule.
- **Ureteric bud**, which is an outgrowth of the mesonephric duct (this eventually dilates and splits to form the renal pelvis, calyces and collecting tubules).

The mesonephric tissue forms a cap over the ureteric bud (ampulla), which grows towards the metanephric blastoma, dilates and divides repeatedly. This eventually forms the pelvis, the major and minor calcyces and the collecting ducts of the kidneys. The ampulla differentiates into the nephron once fusion with the metanephric blastema is complete. A solid clump of cells near the differentiating ampulla is converted into a vesicle and fuses with the ampulla, to eventually become a web of capillaries known as the glomerulus.

The metanephros initially relies on the pelvic branches of the aorta for its blood supply. Later on, the kidney ascends to the lumbar region and its primary blood supply is from the renal arteries, which branch from the aorta. Finally, the hilum of the kidney rotates from its anterior position to rest medially.

The ureters develop from the part of the ureteric bud between the pelvis and the vesicourethral canal (this develops from part of the hindgut known as the cloaca). They drain into the mesonephric ducts and the urogenital sinus. The urinary bladder develops from the mesoderm, and its epithelium is derived from both the mesoderm (the mesonephric ducts) and the endoderm (vesicourethral canal). This is summarized in Fig. 2.2.

The kidneys and the urinary system both develop from the intermediate mesoderm (at the back of the fetal abdominal cavity).

General organization of the kidneys

Macroscopic organization

The anatomy of the kidneys is shown in Fig. 2.3. The relationships of the kidneys are as follows:

- **Anterior** (Fig. 2.4)**:** to the right kidney: liver, 2nd part of the duodenum and the colon; to the left kidney: stomach, pancreas, spleen, jejunum and descending colon.
- **Posterior:** diaphragm, quadratus lumborum, psoas, 12th rib and three nerves (subcostal, iliohypogastric and ilioinguinal).
- **Medial:** hilum (a deep fissure containing the renal vessels, nerves, lymphatics and the renal pelvis); to the left kidney: aorta; to the right kidney: inferior vena cava.
- **Superior:** adrenal gland.

The kidneys lie in a fatty cushion (perinephric fat) contained within the renal fascia. They have three capsular layers:

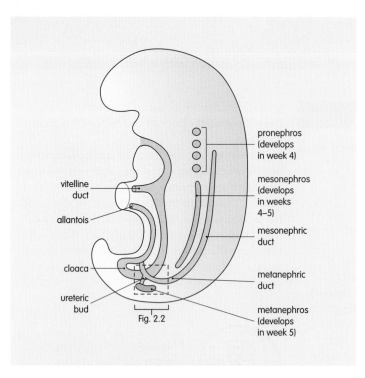

Fig. 2.1 The three embryological renal systems: pronephros, mesonephros and metanephros.

pronephros (develops in week 4)

mesonephros (develops in weeks 4–5)

mesonephric duct

vitelline duct

allantois

cloaca

ureteric bud

metanephric duct

Fig. 2.2

metanephros (develops in week 5)

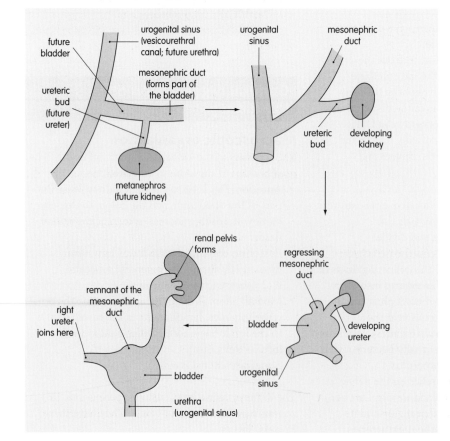

future bladder

urogenital sinus (vesicourethral canal; future urethra)

urogenital sinus

mesonephric duct

ureteric bud (future ureter)

mesonephric duct (forms part of the bladder)

ureteric bud

developing kidney

metanephros (future kidney)

renal pelvis forms

regressing mesonephric duct

remnant of the mesonephric duct

right ureter joins here

bladder

developing ureter

bladder

urogenital sinus

urethra (urogenital sinus)

Fig. 2.2 Development of the kidneys, ureters and bladder.

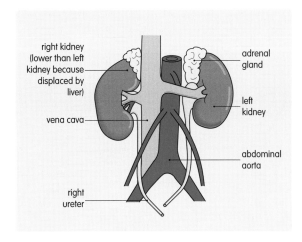

Fig. 2.3 Anatomy of the kidneys.

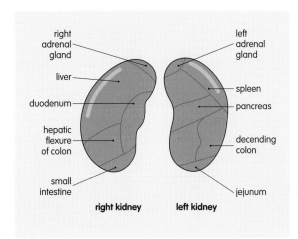

Fig. 2.4 Anterior relations of the kidney.

1. Fascial (renal fascia).
2. Fatty (perinephric fascia).
3. True (fibrous capsule).

Morphology and internal structure

Within the kidney, the ureter continues as the renal pelvis, which lies in a deep fissure called the hilum. The outer border of the renal pelvis divides into two or three major divisions (calyces). These subdivide into a number of minor calyces and are each indented by a papilla of renal tissue called the renal pyramid. It is here that the collecting tubules empty the urine. Along with the renal pelvis, the renal artery, vein, nerve and lymphatics all enter the medial border of the kidney at the hilum (Fig. 2.5).

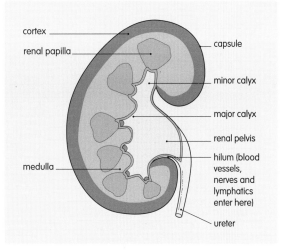

Fig. 2.5 Longitudinal section showing the macroscopic organization of the kidney.

The kidney is divided into two main layers:
1. Outer renal cortex (dark).
2. Inner renal medulla (paler).

The glomeruli in the cortex give it a granular appearance on histology.

The blood supply to the kidneys is from the right and left renal arteries, which branch directly off the abdominal aorta at the level of L1–2. The renal veins drain from the kidneys directly into the vena cava. Lymphatics drain to the para-aortic lymph nodes. The kidney is innervated by sympathetic fibres mainly from the coeliac plexus.

Nephrons

Each kidney has approximately one million nephrons. The nephron (Fig. 2.6) is the functional unit of the kidney and consists of:
1. A renal corpuscle (Bowman's capsule and the glomerulus).
2. Tubule (proximal tubule, loop of Henle, distal tubule and collecting duct).

There are two types of nephron, depending on the length of the loop of Henle:
1. **Cortical nephrons:** these have renal corpuscles in the outer part of the cortex, with a correspondingly short loop of Henle.
2. **Juxtamedullary nephrons:** these have larger renal corpuscles in the inner third of the cortex, with long loops of Henle extending into the medulla.

15

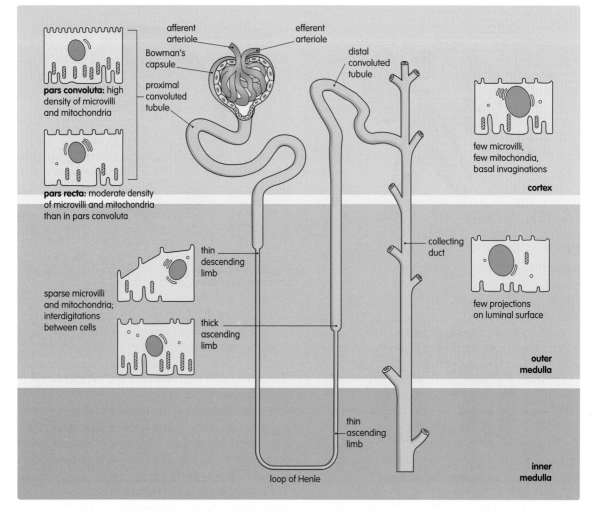

pars convoluta: high density of microvilli and mitochondria

pars recta: moderate density of microvilli and mitochondria than in pars convoluta

afferent arteriole

Bowman's capsule

proximal convoluted tubule

efferent arteriole

distal convoluted tubule

few microvilli, few mitochondia, basal invaginations

cortex

sparse microvilli and mitochondria; interdigitations between cells

thin descending limb

thick ascending limb

collecting duct

few projections on luminal surface

outer medulla

thin ascending limb

inner medulla

loop of Henle

Fig. 2.6 The structure of a nephron and the main histological features of the different cell types within it.

In the human kidney, 85% of the nephrons are cortical nephrons and the remaining 15% are juxtamedullary nephrons.

Glomerulus

The glomerulus is formed by the invagination of a ball of capillaries into the Bowman's capsule, which is the blind end of a nephron. It has a diameter of approximately 200μm.

The function of the glomerulus is to produce a protein-free filtrate from the blood in the glomerular capillaries. The capillaries are supplied by the afferent arterioles and drained by the efferent arterioles. The filtration membrane of the renal corpuscle is made up of three layers and is fundamental to kidney function.

Proximal tubule

The proximal tubule continues from the renal corpuscle. It is 15mm long and 55μm in diameter. Its wall is composed of a single layer of cuboidal cells, which interdigitate extensively and are connected by tight junctions at their luminal surfaces. The luminal edge of each cell is made up of millions of microvilli, forming a dense brush border that increases the surface area available for absorption of tubular filtrate. At the base of each cell there are infoldings of the cell membrane (see Fig. 2.6). The extracellular space between the cells is known as the lateral intercellular space.

The structure of the proximal tubule varies along its length:

- The first part is convoluted (pars convoluta) and cells have an increased density of microvilli and a greater number of mitochondria than cells in the second straight part. This suggests a role in transport of substances across the lumen and the filtrate.
- The second straight part (pars recta) leads on to the first part of the loop of Henle (the thin descending limb).

Loop of Henle

The loop of Henle consists of a single layer of flattened squamous cells, which form a thin-walled, hairpin-shaped tube. The cells of the thin descending segment interdigitate sparingly and have few mitochondria and microvilli on the luminal surface (see Fig. 2.6). This segment ends at the tip of the hairpin loop.

The thin ascending segment is 2 mm long and 20 μm in diameter. Its structure is similar to the preceding part of the tubule (the pars recta), except that the cells have extensive interdigitations. This might have a role in the active transport and permeability properties of the cells. There is an abrupt transition between the thin and thick ascending segments and the level of this depends upon the length of the loop.

The thick ascending segment is 12 mm in length and consists of a single layer of columnar cells. The luminal membrane is invaginated to form many projections, although there is no brush border and there are few infoldings of the basal membrane.

Distal tubule

The distal convoluted tubule is the continuation of the loop of Henle into the cortex, ending in the collecting ducts. The cells have very few microvilli, no brush border and basal infoldings surrounding mitochondria that gradually decrease towards the collecting ducts (see Fig. 2.6). The basal membranes have Na^+/K^+ ATPase pump activity (see p. 26).

Different cell types in this part of the tubule include:
- **Principal cells (P cells):** these contain few mitochondria and respond to antidiuretic hormone (ADH)—also known as vasopressin.
- **Intercalated cells (I cells):** these contain lots of mitochondria and secrete hydrogen ions (H^+).

Collecting ducts

The cortical collecting ducts are 20 mm long. They are lined with cuboidal cells that have a few projections on the luminal surface (see Fig. 2.6). The ducts pass through the renal cortex and medulla and, at the apices of the renal pyramids, drain the urine into the renal pelvis. The renal pelvis is lined by transitional epithelium.

In the cortex each collecting duct drains approximately six distal tubules. In the medulla the distal tubules join together in pairs to form ducts of Bellini and from here drain into the renal calyx.

Renal function and urine formation depends on three basic processes:
- Glomerular filtration.
- Tubular reabsorption.
- Tubular secretion.

Blood supply and vascular structure

The kidneys receive 20–25% of the total cardiac output (1.2 L/min) via the right and left renal arteries. These branch to form interlobar arteries, which further divide to form the arcuate arteries (located at the junction between the cortex and medulla). The interlobular arteries arise at 90 degrees to the arcuate arteries through the cortex, dividing up to form the afferent arterioles. These form glomerular capillary networks and come together to form the efferent arterioles.

The efferent arterioles drain blood from the glomerular capillaries and act as portal vessels (i.e. carry blood from one capillary network to another).
- In the outer two-thirds of the cortex the efferent arterioles form a network of peritubular capillaries that supplies all cortical parts of the nephron.
- In the inner third of the cortex the efferent arterioles follow a hairpin course to form a capillary network surrounding the loops of Henle and the collecting ducts down into the medulla. These vessels are known as the vasa recta.

The vasa recta and the peritubular capillaries drain into the left and right renal veins and then into the inferior vena cava. The microcirculation of the kidney is illustrated in Fig. 2.7.

Fig. 2.7 Organization of the blood circulation within the kidney.

Whilst the peritubular network provides enough oxygen for the cortical nephrons, the medullary supply is only adequate due to the extra blood supplied by the vasa recta.

Function of the renal blood supply

The high rate of blood flow through the kidney is very important in maintaining the homeostatic functions of the kidney. The blood flow through the kidney determines the filtration rate. The oxygen consumption of the kidney is 18mL/min—50% of which is involved in Na^+ reabsorption in the tubules. The vasa recta helps deliver oxygen and nutrients to the nephron segments, and allows the return of reabsorbed substances into the circulation.

Although there is a very substantial blood flow, the arteriovenous oxygen difference is only about

15mL/L, compared with 62mL/L in the brain and 114mL/L in the heart. This means that the oxygen extraction in the kidney is not as efficient as in other organs as a result of shunting of blood in the vasa recta through its hairpin structure.

Juxtaglomerular apparatus (JGA)

The JGA (Fig. 2.8) is located where the thick ascending loop of Henle passes back up into the cortex and lies adjacent to the renal corpuscle and arterioles of its own nephron. It is the area of distal tubule associated with arterioles. The tunica media in the wall of the afferent arteriole contains an area of specialized thickened cells (granular cells), which secrete renin. The epithelium of the distal tubule forms specialized macula densa cells that respond to changes in the composition of the tubular fluid, especially the concentration of sodium ions ($[Na^+]$) in the filtrate. Extraglomerular mesangial cells (Goormaghtigh cells) or lacis cells are found outside the glomerulus, in association with the glomerular apparatus. They are contractile cells identical to the mesangial cells.

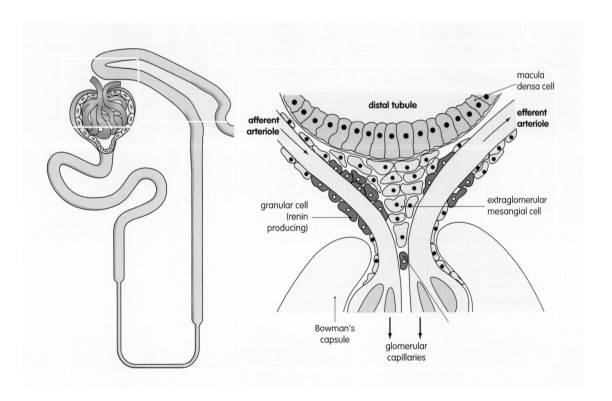

Fig. 2.8 Histology of the juxtaglomerular apparatus.

Hormones produced by the kidney
Renin
Renin is a protein that acts on angiotensinogen to form angiotensin I, which in turn is converted to angiotensin II. Angiotensin II is a potent vasoconstrictor affecting blood pressure, tubular reabsorption of Na^+, and aldosterone secretion from the adrenal glands. Renin release is stimulated by sympathetic stimulation of the granular cells or a decrease in filtrate Na^+ concentration. The latter can occur following a fall in plasma volume, vasodilation of the afferent arterioles and renal ischaemia.

Erythropoietin (EPO)
The kidney is the major source (85%) of EPO production in the adult; in fetal life the liver also produces EPO. It is produced by the peritubular interstitium and the cells of the inner cortex. EPO-sensitive cells are the erythrocyte stem cells found in the bone marrow and the effect of the hormone is to increase the production of erythrocytes, resulting in an increase in the oxygen-carrying capacity of the blood. The half-life of EPO is 5h.

Clinical use of EPO
Hypoxia, anaemia and renal ischaemia all stimulate EPO synthesis (this is a prostaglandin-mediated response). Increased secretion is seen in polycystic kidney disease and renal cell carcinoma, resulting in polycythaemia. Patients with chronic renal failure often have inappropriately low EPO secretion, resulting in normochromic normocytic anaemia. Administration of recombinant EPO (either intravenous or subcutaneous) will correct the anaemia of chronic renal failure.

Vitamin D
Vitamin D is a steroid hormone obtained in the diet, synthesized in the skin from 7-dehydrocholesterol in the presence of sunlight. This naturally occurring vitamin D (cholecalciferol) is hydroxylated in the liver to form 25-hydroxycholecalciferol $(25(OH)D_3)$. It is further hydroxylated in the proximal tubules under the influence of the enzyme 1α-hydroxylase to form the active metabolite 1,25-dihydroxycholecalciferol $(1,25(OH)_2D_3)$. Production of $1,25(OH)_2D_3$ is regulated by parathyroid hormone (PTH), phosphate, and by negative feedback. Active vitamin D is essential for the mineralization of bones and promotes the absorption of calcium ions (Ca^{2+}) and phosphate from the gut.

Glomerular structure and function

Structure of the glomerular filter
The first stage of urine production is the filtration of plasma through the glomerular capillary wall into the Bowman's capsule. The composition of the plasma ultrafiltrate depends on the filtration barrier, which has three layers (Fig. 2.9):
1. The endothelial cells of the glomerular capillary.
2. A basement membrane.
3. The epithelial cells of Bowman's capsule.

Endothelial cells
The endothelial cells lining the glomerular capillaries are thin and flat with large nuclei. The cells are perforated by numerous fenestrae (pores), which have a diameter of 60nm. This allows plasma components to cross the vessel wall, but not blood cells or platelets.

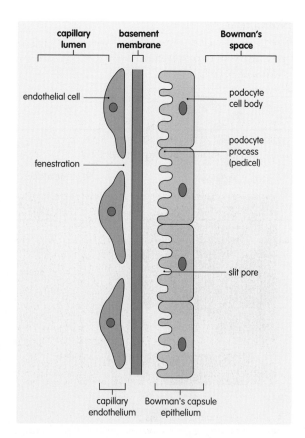

Fig. 2.9 Microscopic organization of the glomerular capillary membrane.

Basement membrane
The basement membrane is a continuous layer of connective tissue and glycoproteins. It is a non-cellular structure that prevents any large molecules from being filtered.

Epithelial lining
The epithelial lining of Bowman's capsule is a single layer of cells (podocytes), which rest on the basement membrane. The podocytes have large extensions or trabeculae, which extend out from the cell body and are embedded in the basement membrane surrounding a capillary. Small processes called pedicels extend out from the trabeculae and interdigitate extensively with the pedicels of adjacent trabeculae. This leads to the formation of slit pores, which control the movement of substances through the final layer of the filter. The podocytes have a well-developed Golgi apparatus, used to produce and maintain the glomerular basement membrane. Podocytes can also be involved in phagocytosis of macromolecules (Figs 2.9 and 2.10).

Mesangium
The mesangium is also part of the renal corpuscle and consists of two components:
1. Mesangial cells.
2. Mesangial matrix.

The mesangial cells surround the glomerular capillaries and have a function similar to monocytes. They provide structural support for the capillaries,

exhibit phagocytic activity, secrete extracellular matrix, and secrete prostaglandins. The cells are contractile, which helps regulate bloodflow through the glomerular capillaries (Fig. 2.11).

Process of glomerular filtration
Filtration of macromolecules depends upon molecular weight, shape and electrical charge. It is a passive process that involves the flow of a solvent through a filter; any molecules that are small enough to pass through the filter form the filtrate. The glomerular filter allows only low-molecular-weight substances in plasma to pass through it, forming the glomerular ultrafiltrate.

Glomerular filtration rate (GFR)
The GFR is the amount of filtrate that is produced from the blood flowing through the glomerulus per unit time.
- Normal GFR is 90–120mL/min/1.73m^2 (i.e. corrected for body surface area).
- The total amount filtered is 180L/day.

The glomerular filtrate normally:
- Contains no blood cells or platelets.
- Contains virtually no protein.
- Is composed mostly of organic solutes with a low molecular weight, and of inorganic ions.

Molecular size
Molecular weight is the main factor in determining whether a substance is filtered or remains in the

Fig. 2.10 Electron micrographs to show the arrangement of podocytes and glomerular capillaries as seen from Bowman's capsule. (A) Processes of podocytes run from the cell body (cb) towards the capillaries where they ultimately split into foot processes (pedicels). (B) Inner surface of a glomerular capillary (from Koeppen BM, Stanton B 1996 Renal physiology, 2nd edn. Mosby Year Book).

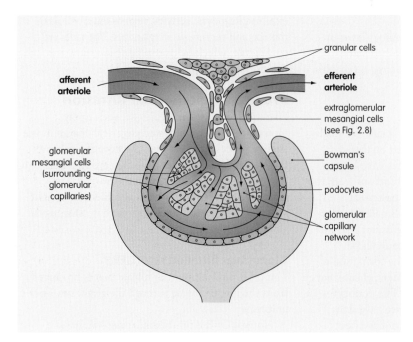

Fig. 2.11 Location of extraglomerular and glomerular mesangial cells.

capillaries. The maximum molecular weight of substances able to pass through the filter is 70kDa. Any molecule with a molecular weight of less than 70kDa passes freely through the filter (e.g. glucose, amino acids, Na^+, urea, K^+). The shape and electrochemical charge of macromolecules also affect filterability. All three layers of the filter are coated with anions and these repel negatively charged macromolecules like albumin. Smaller, positively charged molecules pass through the filtration barriers relatively easily, unless they are protein bound.

Forces governing tissue fluid formation

The movement of fluid between plasma and tissue fluid is determined by Starling's forces (Fig. 2.12):
- Hydrostatic pressure (due to water).
- Colloid osmotic (oncotic) pressure (due to protein).

Changes in these forces alters the GFR.
The following factors affect tissue fluid formation:
- At the arteriole end of the capillary, hydrostatic pressure is greater than colloid oncotic pressure as a result of resistance to flow due to the narrowing of the vessel, and fluid is forced out of the capillary—point 1 in Fig. 2.12A.

- As the fluid moves out of capillaries via the highly permeable wall, oncotic pressure increases and the pressure forces are reversed (most apparent at the venous end of the capillary) so there is net movement of fluid back into the capillaries—point 2 in Fig. 2.12A.

Forces governing GFR

GFR is also driven by Starling forces. However, in the renal vascular bed the surface area of the glomerular capillaries is much larger than that of normal capillary beds, so there is less resistance to flow. The hydrostatic pressure falls less along the length of the capillary because the efferent arterioles, which act as secondary resistance vessels, maintain a constant pressure along the entire length of the glomerular capillary—point 3 in Fig. 2.12B.

Tissue fluid in a vascular bed is the equivalent of glomerular filtrate in Bowman's space, produced as a result of the glomerular capillary hydrostatic pressure (50mmHg). This is opposed by the hydrostatic pressure in Bowman's capsule (12mmHg) and the colloid oncotic pressure (25mmHg) within the capillary. When these forces are equal the filtration equilibrium is reached, with very little fluid movement after this.

Fig. 2.12 Forces involved in tissue fluid formation in a non-renal (A) and a renal (B) vascular bed (see text for detailed explanation).

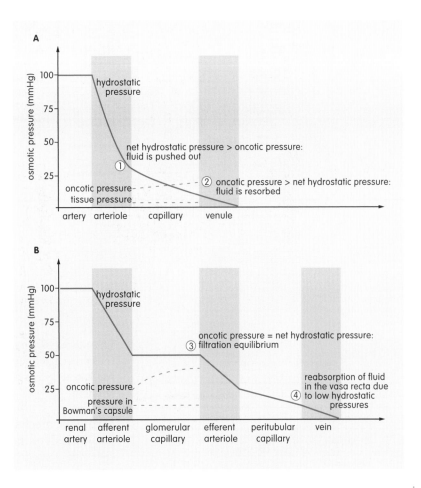

Fluid is reabsorbed into the peritubular capillaries—point 4 in Fig. 2.12B—as a result of high colloid oncotic pressure (35 mmHg) and low hydrostatic pressure. This reabsorption causes a fall in colloid oncotic pressure as plasma proteins become diluted.

The pressures controlling glomerular filtration into Bowman's capsule are illustrated in Fig. 2.13 and the composition of the glomerular filtrate is shown in Fig. 2.14.

Albumin has a molecular weight of 69 kDa and is a negatively charged protein. Only very tiny amounts pass through the glomerular filter because of the repelling effect of its negative charge, and all of this is reabsorbed in the proximal tubule. A total of 30 g of protein a day enters the renal lymph vessels. Significant amounts of protein in the urine (proteinuria) indicates disease in the urinary tract.

Feedback control of glomerular filtration

There are two main mechanisms:
1. **Tubuloglomerular feedback:** this responds to changes in tubular fluid flow rate.
2. **Myogenic mechanism:** this responds to changes in arterial pressure.

Tubuloglomerular feedback mechanism

The GFR remains constant over a wide range of arterial pressures. Because the flow through the capillaries determines the GFR, autoregulation exists within the renal circulation. The tubuloglomerular feedback mechanism controls the GFR of each nephron by sensing the composition of the distal tubular fluid. The system has three components:
1. A luminal component that recognizes a specific variable within the tubular fluid—e.g. the macula

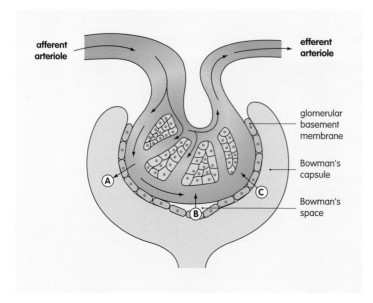

Fig. 2.13 Pressures controlling glomerular filtration into Bowman's capsule. A, Hydrostatic pressure of glomerular capillary = 50mmHg; B, hydrostatic pressure in Bowman's space = 12mmHg (increases fluid uptake into capillary); C, oncotic pressure of glomerular capillary = 25mmHg (increases fluid uptake into capillary).

Labels: afferent arteriole; efferent arteriole; glomerular basement membrane; Bowman's capsule; Bowman's space

Composition of glomerular filtrate	
Component	**Glomerular filtrate**
Na^+ (mmol/L)	142
K^+ (mmol/L)	4.0
Cl^- (mmol/L)	113
HCO_3^- (mmol/L)	28–30
glucose (mmol/L)	5.9
protein (g/100 mL)	0.02

Fig. 2.14 Composition of glomerular filtrate.

densa cells of the tubular epithelium, which detect osmolality or the rate of Na^+ or Cl^- movement into the cells. The higher the flow of the filtrate the higher the Na^+ concentration in the cells.

2. A signal, which is sent via the juxtaglomerular cells, is triggered by a change in the NaCl concentration of distal tubular fluid.
3. An effector (angiotensin II or prostaglandins—refer to chapter 3), which acts as a vasoconstrictor to contract the smooth muscle of the adjacent afferent arterioles and therefore decreases renal plasma flow, which in turn reduces GFR.

This mechanism maintains a constant GFR, thus preventing nephron overload because a high NaCl load decreases the filtration capacity of that nephron.

Myogenic mechanism
This depends on the contraction of smooth muscle cells in response to stretching. Thus, when the arterial pressure rises, the renal afferent arteriole stretches and the smooth muscle cells contract. This prevents the rise in pressure being transmitted to the glomerular capillary, so that the GFR remains unchanged.

Autoregulation of glomerular filitration relies on changes in resistance, primarily in the afferent arterioles.

Transport processes in the renal tubule

The ultrafiltrate produced from the glomerular filter has a similar composition to plasma and is modified by reabsorption and secretion within the tubule to produce the final urine.

Definitions

Reabsorption, secretion and excretion are defined as follows:

- **Reabsorption:** the movement of a substance from the tubular fluid back into the circulation.
- **Secretion:** the movement of substances from the blood into the tubular fluid via tubular cells (active transport) or intercellular spaces (passive process).
- **Excretion:** the removal of waste products from the blood and the net result of filtration, secretion and reabsorption of a substance.

Fig. 2.15 illustrates the processes that occur in the nephron and result in excretion of a substance. Two types of solute transport are involved:

1. Paracellular movement (between cells) across the tight junctions that connect the cells. This is driven by concentration and the electrical and osmotic gradients.
2. Transcellular movement (through cells) via both the apical and basal membranes and the cell cytoplasm. Here, water follows the movement of solutes by osmosis.

Transport mechanisms
Diffusion

Diffusion is the movement of substances down their electrochemical gradient. It is a 'passive' process, as it does not require any metabolic energy or carrier molecules.

Facilitated diffusion

Like diffusion, this is also passive movement of substances along their electrochemical gradient, but it relies on a carrier molecule to transport substances across the membrane. Consequently, it is much faster than diffusion.

Primary active transport

This is an energy-dependent process in which substances cross cell membranes against their concentration and electrochemical gradients. It involves the hydrolysis of adenosine triphosphate (ATP), which provides chemical energy for the transport mechanism.

The most important active transporter is the Na^+/K^+ ATPase pump, which is found on the basal and basolateral membranes of tubular cells. It is involved in the active transport of Na^+ from intracellular to extracellular spaces, allowing the nephron to reabsorb over 99% of the filtered Na^+. This maintains a low Na^+ concentration and a high K^+ concentration in the cell (Fig. 2.16). The other primary active transporters on the tubular cell membrane are:

- Ca^{2+} ATPase.
- H^+/K^+ ATPase.
- H^+ ATPase.

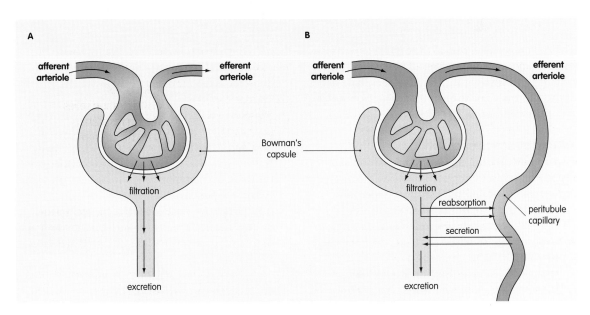

Fig. 2.15 Processes that result in the excretion of a substance in the nephron.

Fig. 2.16 Mechanisms of active transport in the proximal tubule cells:
• H^+/K^+ ATPase
• proton pump
• Ca^{2+} ATPase
• Na^+/K^+ ATPase (sodium pump).

The ATP molecule is part of the protein structure in the primary active transporters. Energy is derived from the hydrolysis of the terminal phosphate bond of the ATP molecule to form adenosine diphosphate (ADP) and phosphate (P_i) (Fig. 2.17).

Secondary active transport

This process uses the energy produced from another process for transporting molecules (i.e. the transport of the solutes is coupled). The most important example of this mechanism involves the Na^+/K^+ ATPase pump as the driving force for the secretion and reabsorption of other solutes in which the energy is provided by the Na^+ gradient.

The Na^+/K^+ ATPase pump creates an ionic gradient across the cell membrane, which allows the energy produced from the diffusion of Na^+ into the cell as it moves along its electrochemical gradient to be used for active transport (i.e. against their electrochemical gradients) of other solutes.

Substances can move in two directions by the following processes:

• **Symport:** energy produced by the movement of Na^+ is used to transport other substances in the same direction across the cell membrane—i.e. with the Na^+ gradient (e.g. the $Na^+/K^+/Cl^-$ cotransporter in the thick ascending limb and the Na^+/glucose in the cells of the proximal tubule cells).

• **Antiport:** movement of substances against their electrochemical gradient in the opposite direction to the Na^+ gradient (e.g. the Ca^{2+}/Na^+ and the H^+/Na^+ exchangers).

These processes are carried out by specific carrier proteins embedded in the cell membrane called transporters.

Ion channels

These are protein pores found on the epithelial cell membranes. They allow rapid transport of ions into the cell. Channels that are specific for Na^+, K^+ and Cl^- are found on the apical membrane of all the cells lining the nephron. Although transport through these channels is very fast (10^6–10^8 ions/s) there are only about 100 channels per cell, compared with the slower (100 ions/s) but more numerous active transporters (10^7 transporters per cell).

blocked by digitalis

outside cell

cell membrane

intracellular

$3Na^+$ $2K^+$

β

α

β

α

stimulated by
high intracellular
$[Na^+]$ ATP   ADP + P_i

$3Na^+$ $2K^+$

Fig. 2.17 Na^+/K^+ ATPase pump found in the basal membrane of the cells. It drives secondary active transport by maintaining a low Na^+ concentration in the cells.

Handling of sodium by the kidney

Na^+ ions can be used to show how the filtrate is modified by various regions of the nephron to produce the excreted urine. The concentration of Na^+ in the Bowman's capsule is equal to the plasma level because Na^+ is freely filtered. Virtually all the Na^+ that is filtered into the nephron is reabsorbed back into the circulation, with only 1% or less of the filtered Na^+ being excreted in the urine. This is important not only to preserve Na^+ levels in the body but also because the reabsorption processes of glucose, amino acids, water, lactate, Cl^-, HCO_3^- and PO_4^{3-} ions depend upon the movement of Na^+ back into the cells of the tubule. Na^+ transport along the nephron is shown in Fig. 2.18.

Generating Na^+ gradients within the kidney is central to the reabsorption of many substances, including glucose, amino acids, water, lactate, Cl^-, HCO_3^-, and PO_4^{3-}.

The proximal tubule

Microstructure

The proximal tubule is made up of two parts:
1. Pars convoluta.
2. Pars recta.

Na+ transport along the nephron			
Part of nephron	Percentage of filtered Na+ reabsorbed	Method of entry into the cell	Regulatory hormones
proximal tubule	65–70	Na+ co-transport, paracellular	angiotensin II
loop of Henle	20–25	Na+/Cl−/K+ pump (1:2:1)	aldosterone
early distal tubule	5	Na+/Cl− symport	aldosterone
late distal tubule and collecting ducts	5	Na+ channels	aldosterone, atrial natriuretic peptide

Fig. 2.18 Na^+ transport along the nephron.

The most active transport occurs in the cells of the pars convoluta. The features of a proximal tubule cell are shown in Fig. 2.19. Histology is discussed earlier (see Fig. 2.6).

Transport of sodium and chloride

Movement of sodium into the lateral space

Seventy per cent of the filtered Na^+ is reabsorbed in the proximal tubule. A lot of Na^+ is reabsorbed in the early proximal tubule but, as the cell junctions are leaky, the concentration gradient between the filtrate and the intercellular plasma is limited. Less reabsorption occurs in the late proximal tubule but the cell junctions are tight, so a better concentration gradient is established. The primary transporter Na^+/K^+ ATPase (Na^+ pump) on the basolateral membrane actively transports Na^+ out of the cell into the lateral intercellular spaces between adjacent cells.

Sodium entry into the cell

This movement of Na^+ out of the cell maintains a very low concentration of Na^+ within the proximal tubule cells (less than 30mmol/L). This, and the fact that there is a negative transmembrane potential relative to the lumen (−70mV), drives Na^+ ions to move along their concentration and electrical gradients into the cells from the tubular fluid via carrier molecules on the apical membrane. In the early proximal tubule, movement of other substances is coupled with Na^+ transport in and out of tubule cells:

- Glucose, amino acids, PO_4^{3-} and lactate are transported by symport with Na^+ into the cell.
- H^+ is transported by antiport out of the cell and linked to the reabsorption of HCO_3^-.

In the late proximal tubule, Na^+ is mainly reabsorbed with Cl^- across the cells. This occurs because the cells of the late proximal tubule have different Na^+ transport mechanisms and the tubular fluids have very little glucose and amino acids. The forces governing Na^+ transport in the proximal tubule are shown in Fig. 2.20.

Chloride reabsorption

Over 60% of filtered Cl^- is reabsorbed in the middle and late proximal tubule. Chloride ions enter the cells by passive reabsorption; however, the intercellular potential opposes Cl^- entry into the cells in the early part of the proximal tubule. The reabsorption of glucose, amino acids and HCO_3^- with Na^+ in the initial part of the proximal tubule creates a filtrate that becomes concentrated with Cl^-. The increase in Cl^- produces a diffusion gradient, which allows movement of the ions into the intercellular space or directly into the cell:

Fig. 2.19 Features of a proximal tubule cell.

- Most Cl⁻ entry is via the tight junctions between cells along with Na⁺.
- A small amount of Cl⁻ enters by antiport with HCO_3^- and $HCOO^-$ (formate).

Water reabsorption

Seventy per cent of the filtered water is reabsorbed in the proximal tubule. This is driven by a transtubular osmotic gradient, created by solute reabsorption into the lateral intercellular spaces (Fig. 2.21). This leaves a dilute solution, which causes an increase in the hydrostatic pressure, so fluid moves by osmosis through the basement membrane into the peritubular capillary. This movement is also driven by the high oncotic pressure in the peritubular capillary because of the high

Forces governing Na⁺ transport in the proximal tubule			
Part of proximal tubule	Electrical potential (mV)	Transport mechanism	Na⁺ concentration (mmol/L)
tubular lumen	–2	passive (carrier molecule)	150
cell	–70	active (pump)	30
extracellular fluid	0	diffusion	150

Fig. 2.20 Forces governing Na⁺ transport in the proximal tubule.

Fig. 2.21 Na⁺ transport processes in the proximal tubule.

plasma protein concentration created by the filtration process in the glomerulus.

The fluid leaving the proximal tubule is isosmotic because both ions and water move out of the filtrate together. The proximal tubule has no concentrating capacity.

Transport of other solutes in the proximal tubule

Glucose

Normal plasma glucose concentration is 2.5–5.5 mmol/L. Usually, 0.2–0.5 mmol of glucose is filtered every minute. An increase in the plasma glucose concentration results in a proportional increase in the amount of glucose filtered. Virtually all filtered glucose is reabsorbed in the proximal tubule, unless the amount of filtered glucose exceeds the resorptive capacity of the cells. Glucose is transported into the proximal tubule cells by symport against its concentration gradient. It is driven by the energy released from the transport of Na^+ down its electrochemical gradient because the Na^+/K^+ ATPase pump on the basolateral membrane maintains a low Na^+ concentration and negative potential within the cell (Fig. 2.22). This is an example of secondary active transport. The transport ratio is:

- 1:1 Na^+: glucose in the pars convoluta.
- 2:1 Na^+: glucose in the pars recta.

T_m is the maximum tubular resorptive capacity for a solute (i.e. the point of saturation for the carriers), and this value can be calculated for glucose. All nephrons have different thresholds for

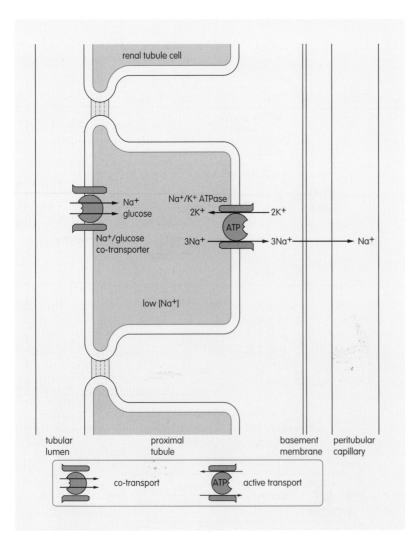

Fig. 2.22 Active transport of glucose in the proximal tubule (pars convoluta). This occurs against a concentration gradient.

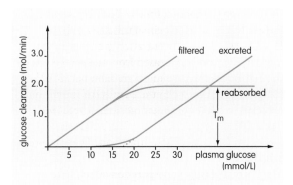

Fig. 2.23 Relationship between plasma concentration, filtration, reabsorption and excretion of glucose (GFR = 100 mL/min). T_m is exceeded in nephrons with plasma glucose >10 mmol/L and for all nephrons when plasma glucose >20 mmol/L (nephron heterogeneity gives rise to 'splay' on the curve).

glucose reabsorption (nephron heterogeneity). There are a limited number of Na^+/glucose carrier molecules, so glucose reabsorption is T_m limited. Fig. 2.23 shows that the lowest renal threshold of glucose is at a plasma glucose concentration of 10 mmol/L. At this level, filtered glucose will begin to be excreted in the urine (glycosuria). If the plasma glucose concentration increases further even those nephrons with highest resorptive capacity become saturated, and glucose is excreted. Urinary glucose increases in parallel with plasma glucose. The T_m for glucose is exceeded in all nephrons when the plasma glucose concentration is >20 mmol/L.

Glycosuria occurs if:
- The filtered load exceeds the renal threshold.
- T_m for glucose is lower than normal.

In diabetes, plasma glucose is elevated, so the filtered load of glucose is increased—if plasma glucose exceeds 10 mmol/L, glycosuria will result. In certain inherited tubular disorders, T_m for glucose is low and glycosuria can be found with a normal plasma glucose (renal glycosuria)—the patient is not diabetic. Renal glycosuria can also occur in pregnancy, because T_m for glucose is reduced; however, it should be noted that true diabetes can also occur in pregnancy and cause glycosuria. A glucose tolerance test can be used to distinguish between the two.

Amino acids
Amino acids are the basic unit of proteins and are absorbed constantly from the gut. The plasma concentration of amino acids is 2.5–3.5 mmol/L.

They are small molecules that filter easily through the glomerulus, with most reabsorption occurring in the proximal tubule. The transport is a secondary active process (by symport with Na^+) and is driven by Na^+/K^+ ATPase, as with glucose. There are at least five different transport systems coupled with Na^+ and these are responsible for the movement of different types of amino acid residue. This is a T_m-limited process, so amino aciduria results if the reabsorption mechanism is saturated or if the reabsorption mechanism is defective (i.e. in Fanconi syndrome).

Phosphate
Phosphate (PO_4^{3-}) salts are essential for the structure of bones and teeth. Eighty per cent of the body's PO_4^{3-} content is in bone and 20% is in the intracellular fluid (ICF). It is filtered easily at the glomerulus; 80% is then reabsorbed in the proximal tubule and the remaining 20% is excreted in urine.

The kidneys play an important role in the regulation of PO_4^{3-}. The amount filtered is proportional to the plasma PO_4^{3-} concentration. Therefore, any increase in plasma PO_4^{3-} concentration (>1.2 mmol/L) leads to an increase in the amount filtered and excreted, which is how plasma PO_4^{3-} levels are controlled. A fall in GFR will result in increased plasma PO_4^{3-} concentration. Reabsorption of PO_4^{3-} occurs with Na^+ ions (two Na^+ for every PO_4^{3-} ion) at the apical membrane of the tubular cells.

PO_4^{3-} is an important urinary buffer for H^+ and its excretion is influenced by:
- Parathyroid hormone (increases excretion).
- Vitamin D (decreases excretion).
- Acidosis (increases excretion).
- Glucocorticoids (increases excretion).

Urea
Urea is the end-product of protein metabolism, which occurs in the liver. Urea is transported to the kidneys via the blood. It is a small molecule that is filtered freely at the glomerulus. The normal plasma concentration of urea is 2.5–7.5 mmol/L. Urea concentration increases in the filtrate as a result of Na^+, Cl^- and water reabsorption. This allows passive reabsorption of 40–50% of urea along its concentration gradient; 50–60% of the filtered urea is excreted in the urine. Antidiuretic hormone (ADH) increases the permeability of the inner medullary collecting ducts to urea. The distal tubule and the outer medullary ducts are impermeable to urea.

Bicarbonate

Bicarbonate (HCO_3^-) is vital for the maintenance of acid–base balance within the body. The plasma concentration of HCO_3^- is 20–30 mmol/L. The kidney plays an important part in pH regulation by controlling the plasma HCO_3^- concentration. The proximal tubule reabsorbs 80% of the filtered HCO_3^- (Fig. 2.24), the remaining 20% being taken up in the distal tubule and collecting ducts. Reabsorption of HCO_3^- is coupled to Na^+ transport.

Mechanism of HCO_3^- reabsorption

Na^+ reabsorption on the apical membrane drives H^+ secretion by the tubular cells. H^+ combines with HCO_3^- ions to form H_2CO_3 (carbonic acid). Carbonic anhydrase (CA) on the brush border of the cells catalyses the dissociation of H_2CO_3 to $H_2O +$ CO_2 within the tubular lumen. Both H_2O and CO_2 diffuse freely into the cell, where they reform H_2CO_3, this process being catalysed by intracellular CA. HCO_3^- and Na^+ are actively transported out of the cell across the basolateral membrane. H^+ is secreted out of the cell into the tubular lumen and recycled to allow continuation of this cycle (see Fig. 2.24).

Sulphate

The normal plasma concentration of sulphate is 1–1.5 mmol/L. Sulphate reabsorption is T_m limited and this is an important mechanism in regulating its plasma concentration.

Potassium

The plasma concentration of potassium is 4–5 mmol/L. Approximately 70% of K^+ is reabsorbed

Fig. 2.24 HCO_3^- reabsorption in the proximal tubule cells. Secreted H^+ combines with HCO_3^- to form carbonic acid. This is broken down by carbonic anhydrase (CA) in the brush border to CO_2 and H_2O, which diffuse freely into the cell. The process is reversed inside the cell to re-form HCO_3^-.

in the proximal tubule, mostly by passive paracellular reabsorption across the tight junctions between tubular cells. K^+ can be secreted or reabsorbed in the nephron. Excretion of the filtered K^+ can vary from 1% to 110% depending on:

- Dietary intake of potassium.
- Acid–base status.
- Aldosterone levels.

K^+ reabsorption occurs mainly in the thick ascending loop of Henle by cotransport of $Na^+/K^+/Cl^-$ on the luminal membrane. Reabsorption of K^+ occurs in the distal tubule during severe dietary depletion of K^+.

The proximal tubule is the primary site for reabsorption of water and solutes.
- In the early proximal tubule, Na^+ is reabsorbed with HCO_3^- and organic ions.
- In the late proximal tubule, Na^+ is reabsorbed with Cl^-.

Secretion by the proximal tubule

Secretion is the movement of solutes from the proximal tubule cells into the tubular fluid. It can be active (i.e. require energy) or passive. These processes are T_m limited or gradient time-limited.

There are three T_m-limited secretory mechanisms for:

1. Strong organic bases (e.g. choline, histamine and thiamine), which are secreted in the pars convoluta.
2. Strong organic acids (e.g. penicillin, *p*-aminohippuric acid—PAH), which are secreted in the pars recta as the substances move out from the peritubular capillaries.
3. Ethylenediaminetetra acetic acid (EDTA).

The substances handled by gradient time-limited mechanisms include:

- H^+: secretion of H^+ depends on the transport of Na^+ and the reabsorption of HCO_3^-. The movement of H^+ out of the cells occurs by an antiport with Na^+ on the apical membrane using a specific transporter.
- K^+: this varies, and depends on diet, aldosterone levels, acid–base status and the urine flow.

Role of the loop of Henle

The loop of Henle reabsorbs 20% of the filtered Na^+ and 15% of tubular water. As filtrate flows through the loop of Henle, reabsorption of NaCl in the thick ascending limb produces a hypertonic interstitial fluid in the surrounding medulla. This creates a concentration gradient and water moves passively out of the thin descending limb.

The tubular fluid is isotonic to the plasma on entering the loop of Henle; however, by the time it leaves the loop it is hypotonic because ion reabsorption occurs within the loop. This mechanism allows urine to be concentrated, using the least amount of energy, because water is then reabsorbed passively from the collecting ducts into the hypertonic interstitium of the medulla.

Structure of the loop of Henle

The different components of the loop are functionally separate units, each with its own specific properties.

Thin descending limb

The thin descending limb is lined by thin, flat cells that have minimal cytoplasmic specialization. It is permeable to water, Na^+ and Cl^-. Water is reabsorbed passively down a concentration gradient caused by the hypertonic interstitium of the medulla. NaCl moves into the lumen and water moves out of the lumen into the interstitium, allowing the tubular fluid to come into equilibrium with the interstitium.

- The juxtamedullary nephrons have long, thin limbs that extend deep into the inner medulla.
- The cortical nephrons only just enter the medulla and some are situated entirely in the cortex.

Thin ascending limb

The thin ascending limb has a similar structure to the thin descending limb but is impermeable to water and has minimal NaCl transport occurring within the cells.

Thick ascending limb

The thick ascending limb consists of large cells with mitochondria, which generate energy for the active transport of Na^+ (20% of filtered Na^+ is reabsorbed in the loop of Henle) and Cl^- ions from the tubular fluid into the interstitium. As a result, the filtrate becomes progressively diluted (this part of the tubule is impermeable to water). There is cotransport (symport) of Na^+, Cl^- and K^+ (in the ratio 1:2:1—so the pump is electrochemically neutral) on the apical membrane. This transport process is driven by the Na^+ gradient across the cell membrane. Na^+ is removed from the cell by the Na^+/K^+ ATPase pump on the basolateral membrane and K^+ and Cl^- diffuse passively out as a result of Na^+ movement; however, most of the K^+ leaks back into the cell and tubular lumen. Overall, NaCl accumulates in the medullary interstitium. Figure 2.25 shows the transport processes in the loop of Henle; the inset shows the transport of ions in the cells in the thick ascending limb of the loop of Henle.

Countercurrent multiplication

Any mechanism that will concentrate urine must be able to reabsorb water from the tubular fluid as it passes through the collecting ducts. The loop of Henle, which acts as a countercurrent multiplier, produces a hypertonic medulla by pooling NaCl in the interstitium, which favours the subsequent movement of water out of the collecting ducts (under the regulation of ADH). Each portion of the loop contributes to the effectiveness of this system.

The mechanism of the countercurrent multiplier is illustrated in Fig 2.26.

The thick, ascending limb can maintain a difference of $200 mOsmol/kgH_2O$ between the tubular fluid and the interstitium at any point along its length. The maximum osmolality of the interstitium is $1400 mOsmol/kgH_2O$ (normal plasma osmolality is $300 mOsmol/kgH_2O$) at the tip of the loop. The fluid leaving the loop of Henle is hypotonic ($100 mOsmol/kgH_2O$).

Role of urea and vasa recta

The countercurrent mechanism requires an environment in which the waste products and water are cleared without disturbing the solutes that maintain the medullary hypertonicity. This exchange is provided by the vasa recta capillary system derived from the efferent arterioles of the longer juxtaglomerular nephrons. It does not require metabolic energy.

The capillaries have a hairpin arrangement surrounding the loop of Henle and are permeable to water and solutes. As the descending vessels pass through the medulla they absorb solutes such as Na^+, urea and Cl^-. Water moves along its osmotic gradient out of the capillaries. At the tip of the loop the capillary blood has the same osmolality as the interstitium, and an osmotic equilibrium is reached. The capillaries that ascend with the corresponding loop of Henle contain very viscous concentrated blood as a result of the earlier loss of water from the capillaries. There is a consequent increase in oncotic pressure because of the concentration of plasma proteins, which favours the movement of water back into the blood vessel from the interstitium. However, most of the NaCl is retained in the interstitium to maintain the hypertonic medullary environment.

The collecting tubules pass through the cortex and medulla. They consist of two functionally different parts:
1. The cortical collecting ducts.
2. The medullary (inner and outer) collecting ducts.

Both parts are impermeable to NaCl. The permeability to water and urea (only in the inner medullary collecting ducts) varies according to the presence of antidiuretic hormone (ADH). ADH increases the permeability to water and thus controls the concentration of the urine produced. ADH acts to increase water uptake in the cortical collecting tubules resulting in the production of a more concentrated urine.

The water reabsorbed in the medullary part of the collecting ducts is taken up by the vasa recta to prevent dilution of the medullary interstitium, which is crucial to the function of the distal nephron and the concentration of urine.

Although about 20% of the initial glomerular filtrate enters the distal nephron, only 5% enters the medullary collecting ducts. This is mainly due to water reabsorption in the cortical tubules.

The structure, location and function of the loop of Henle has a central role in the development of a hypertonic gradient in the medulla. This allows urine to be concentrated as it passes through the collecting tubules.

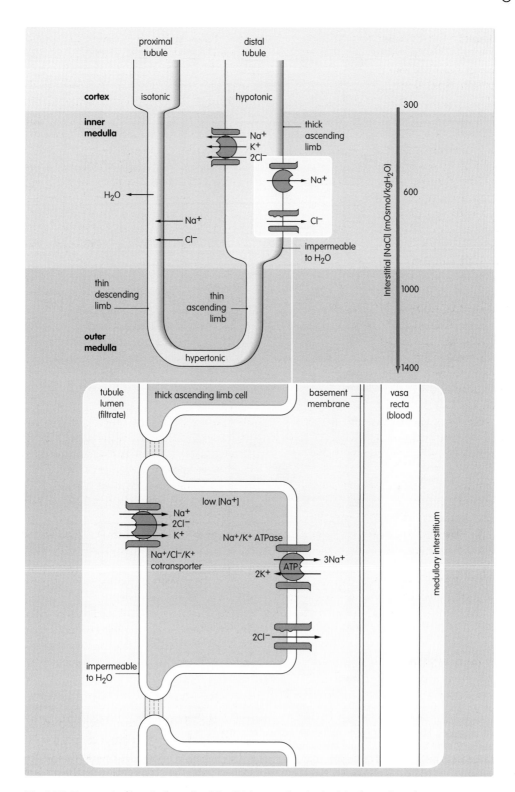

Fig. 2.25 Transport of ions in the cells of the thick ascending limb of the loop of Henle:
• Na⁺/Cl⁻/K⁺ cotransporter
• Na⁺/K⁺ ATPase
• Cl⁻ channel.

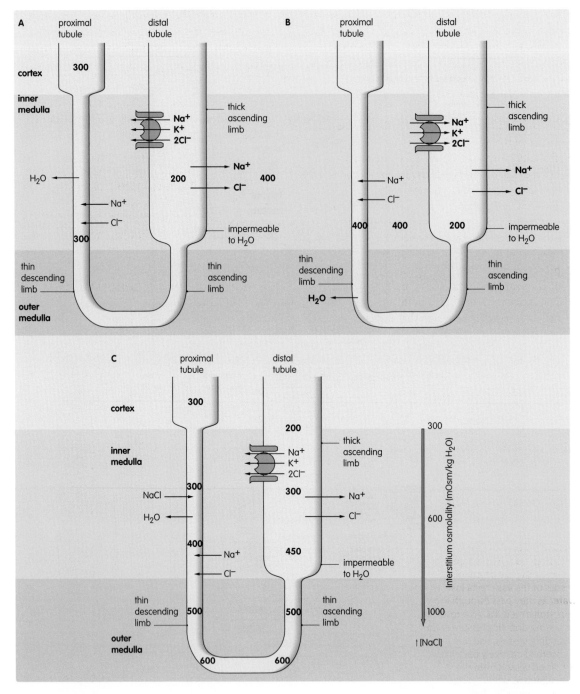

Fig. 2.26 (A) As active reabsorption of Na^+, Cl^- and K^+ occurs in the thick ascending limb, the concentration of solutes in the medulla increases. Because there is no movement of water in the thick ascending limb, the osmolality of the tubular fluid decreases ($200\,mOsmol/kgH_2O$) and the osmolality of the interstitium increases ($400\,mOsmol/kgH_2O$).

(B) The increase in the interstitial osmolality stimulates passive movement of water out of the thin descending limb into the medullary interstitium. It also causes NaCl to move into the filtrate. This occurs until an equilibrium is reached ($400\,mOsmol/kgH_2O$) between the thin descending limb and the interstitium.

(C) The constant removal of NaCl will continue to decrease the osmolality of the tubular fluid in the thick ascending limb, with maximal reabsorption occurring at the tip of the loop ($600\,mOsmol/kgH_2O$). This will further increase the osmolality of the fluid in the thin descending limb as it comes into equilibrium with its surroundings. In this way, a longitudinal gradient of osmolality is created in the medulla.

Figure 2.27 shows the countercurrent exchanger and the collecting duct as it passes through the medulla.

Although urea is impermeable in the cortical collecting tubules, ADH affects the permeability of urea within the medullary cortical tubules. Urea, along with NaCl, helps maintain medullary hypertonicity as follows:

- 50% of the filtered urea is reabsorbed in the proximal tubule with Na^+.
- The tubular concentration of urea increases as it diffuses out of the medullary interstitium into the lumen down its concentration gradient.
- The remaining urea becomes further concentrated within the tubular lumen as water and other solutes are reabsorbed into the cells of the distal tubule and the cortical collecting tubules, a process aided by the fact that these parts of the nephron are impermeable to urea.
- The concentration of urea in the medullary collecting tubules is so high that it diffuses out of

the lumen into the interstitium, thus increasing the concentration of urea in the medulla and recycling it. This occurs in the presence of ADH.

A high-protein diet increases the amount of urea in the blood for excretion as a result of increased metabolism. Consequently, there is more urea in the medullary interstitium, resulting in a higher urine osmolality.

Urine concentration and solute content can be altered to match homeostatic demands

Regulation of urine concentration
ADH levels within the body determine the concentration and volume of urine:

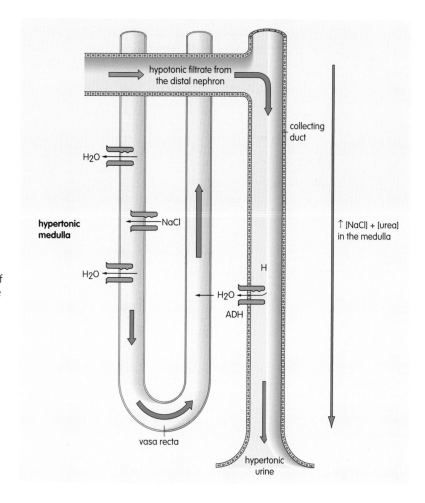

Fig. 2.27 Countercurrent exchanger as it passes through the medulla. The descending vessels of the vasa recta lose water as they pass through the hypertonic medulla. As a result of increasing oncotic pressure in the ascending vessels, water is reabsorbed passively back into the blood vessels from the interstitium as water uptake occurs in the collecting ducts under the influence of ADH. Because of this uptake of water by the vasa recta, the high osmolality of the medullary interstitium is maintained and this hypertonic environment allows continued concentration of the tubular fluid in the collecting duct.

- Average daily urine volume is 1.0–1.5L (normal range 400mL to 2–3L).
- Average urine osmolality is 450mOsmol/kgH$_2$O (normal range 60–1400mOsmol/kgH$_2$O).

The presence of cortisol is vital for the action of ADH. Aldosterone is also very important in concentrating urine because it affects Na$^+$ reabsorption. By increasing Na$^+$ uptake in the cortical collecting tubules more water is passively reabsorbed, so urine volume decreases and osmolality increases (ADH is considered further in Chapter 3).

- Describe the anatomical relations of the right and left kidney.
- Describe the structure of the five anatomical regions of the nephron.
- Name the two different types of nephrons, and give three ways in which they differ.
- List four hormones that act on the kidney and four that are produced by the kidney.
- Discuss how the kidney is involved in vitamin D metabolism.
- Describe the structure of the glomerular filter.
- Explain how the molecular size of particles affects filtration.
- Define reabsorption, secretion and excretion.
- Describe the difference between primary and secondary active transport.
- Outline sodium handling by the proximal tubule.
- Using a graph, explain how glucose reabsorption in the proximal tubule is 'T$_m$ limited'.
- Name two other substances reabsorbed in the proximal tubule whose T$_m$ is also limited.
- Discuss the reabsorption of HCO$_3^-$ in the proximal tubule.
- Summarize the countercurrent mechanism of the loop of Henle.
- Explain how ADH affects urine concentration.

3. Renal Function

Renal blood flow and the glomerular filtration rate (GFR)

Measurement of the GFR
Clearance
Clearance (C) is the volume of plasma that is cleared of a substance in a unit time. It is a measure of the kidney's ability to remove a substance from the plasma and excrete it. The units used are volume and time—usually ml/min. If P_x = concentration of substance x in arterial plasma (mg/mL), U_x = concentration of x in the urine (mg/mL) and V = urine flow rate (mL/min), then the clearance of substance x is:

$$C_x = \frac{U_x \times V}{P_x}$$

Clearance of a substance will provide an accurate estimate of GFR if that substance 'follows' the filtrate without being altered by the kidney (i.e. is not reabsorbed, secreted, synthesized or metabolized by the kidney). Inulin is such a substance:
- It is a polysaccharide of molecular weight 5500.
- It is not normally found within the body, so is introduced into the body by injection or intravenous infusion.
- It passes into the glomerular filtrate but is not reabsorbed, secreted, synthesized or metabolized by the kidney—so all inulin filtered by the glomerulus is excreted in the urine. Inulin clearance can be used to assess glomerular function in disease.

Normal inulin clearance is equal to the GFR, i.e. 120mL/min/1.73m² body surface area (this varies with body size). However, measurement of inulin clearance is complicated and is rarely used to assess GFR in routine clinical practice. Instead, creatinine clearance is used as an estimate of GFR. Creatinine is found in the body; it is produced during muscle metabolism:

$$\text{Phosphocreatine} + \text{ADP} \xrightarrow{\overset{\text{Creatine}}{\text{phosphokinase}}} \text{Creatine} + \text{ATP}$$

$$\text{Creatine} + H_2O \longrightarrow \text{Creatinine}$$

Plasma creatinine levels remain constant if renal function, muscle mass and metabolism are stable. Plasma creatinine is commonly used to indicate renal function. Its exact value depends upon muscle mass and therefore age, sex and size. It has a reciprocal relationship with GFR, which is shown in Fig. 3.1.

Like inulin, creatinine is filtered freely and is not affected or produced by the kidney. It can therefore be used to measure GFR. However, some creatinine is secreted by the tubules, causing it to slightly overestimate the GFR. This is thought to be cancelled out by inaccuracies in the measurement of creatinine, which overestimate the true plasma creatinine concentration.

Clearance ratios
Information about how the kidney clears a particular substance, x (C_x), can be obtained by comparing its clearance with that of inulin (C_{in}):
- Substances with clearance values greater than inulin clearance ($C_x > C_{in}$): the substance enters the renal tubule by glomerular filtration and tubular secretion (e.g. *p*-aminohippuric acid—PAH).
- Substances with clearance values lower than inulin clearance ($C_x < C_{in}$): the substance is either not freely filtered at the glomerulus or is freely filtered, but then reabsorbed from the tubule.

Measurement of renal blood flow
The Fick principle states that the amount of substance x removed from plasma by the kidney in 1 min is equal to the amount appearing in urine in 1 min. This is illustrated by the formula below, where RPF = renal plasma flow, A_x = arterial concentration of a substance, V_x = venous concentration, U_x = urinary concentration and V = urinary flow rate:

$$(A_x - V_x) \times \text{RPF} = V \times U_x$$

PAH is an organic acid that is filtered at the glomerulus and secreted by the proximal tubules (transport maximum (T_m) limited). Thus, the amount of PAH excreted equals the amount filtered and secreted in the kidney. If the T_m for PAH is not

Fig. 3.1 Relationship of plasma creatinine and glomerular filtration rate (GFR). Normal GFR is typically 90–120 mL/min (from Koeppen BM, Stanton B. 1996 Renal physiology, 2nd edn. Mosby Year Book).

Fig. 3.2 Filtration, secretion and excretion of *p*-aminohippuric acid (PAH) compared with its plasma concentration.

exceeded, at least 90% is removed from the blood as it passes through the kidney in a normal individual. Therefore the clearance of PAH can be used to measure RPF (Fig. 3.2). If plasma PAH concentration is less than 0.1 mg/mL, T_m for PAH is not exceeded. The extraction of PAH from the blood approaches 100%, so venous concentration of PAH is zero (V_{PAH}) and C_{PAH} equals renal plasma flow.

When the excretion of PAH is 100%, if P_{PAH} = the plasma concentration of PAH, U_{PAH} = the urine concentration of PAH and V = urinary flow rate:

$$RPF \times P_{PAH} = V \times U_{PAH}$$

or

$$RPF = \frac{V \times U_{PAH}}{P_{PAH}} = C_{PAH}$$

The normal RPF is 600 mL/min.

Renal blood flow (RBF) can be obtained from RPF by using the haematocrit (the percentage of total blood volume that is made of erythrocytes). The haematocrit is 45%, so 55% of blood is made up of plasma:

$$RBF = RPF \times 100/55$$
$$= 600 \times 100/55$$
$$= 1100 \, mL/min$$

However, C_{PAH} is not an exact measurement of RPF. This is because renal blood flows to the capsule, perirenal fat and medulla, as well as to the glomeruli and tubules. Therefore, PAH clearance estimates cortical plasma flow and is usually referred to as effective RPF (ERPF).

If PAH excretion is reduced significantly, C_{PAH} becomes a less reliable marker of RPF unless this is taken into account. Excretion is reduced:

- When [PAH] is greater than T_m.
- In chronic renal failure.
- In tubular dysfunction.

p-aminohippuric acid (PAH) clearance provides a non-invasive estimate of the renal plasma flow.

Other methods of measuring RBF (not used routinely in clinical practice)

Inert gas 'washout' technique

Radioactive krypton (^{84}Kr) or xenon (^{133}Xe) is injected into the renal artery with a small amount of saline. The gas diffuses throughout the kidneys almost immediately, at a rate dependent upon RBF. Therefore, the rate of removal of gas from the kidneys can be used to determine RBF.

Isotope uptake technique

Radioactive potassium (^{42}K) or rubidium (^{86}Rb) is given intravenously. The amount of isotope in different parts of the kidney gives an indication of the blood flow through the kidney. This method

Fig. 3.3 The regulation of renal blood flow (RBF) and glomerular filtration rate (GFR) by vasoconstriction of arterioles.

requires removal of the kidneys and is therefore used only in experimental studies in animals.

Filtration fraction

This is the percentage of plasma flow passing the glomerulus that is filtered:

Filtration fraction = GFR/RPF

In a normal man:

$$\text{Filtration fraction} = 120/600 = 20\%$$

Fractional excretion (FE)

This is a measure of net reabsorption or net secretion of a substance (x):

$$FE_x = \text{mass excreted/mass filtered} = (U_x \times V)/(GFR \times P_x)$$

FE is often expressed as a percentage. Therefore, if the FE is 0.24, 24% of the filtered mass is excreted and 76% undergoes net reabsorption.

Regulation of RBF and GFR

- RBF is 1100mL/min (RPF is 600mL/min).
- GFR is 120mL/min.

Both remain fairly constant because of autoregulation, which involves changes in tone of the afferent and efferent arterioles (Fig. 3.3). Over the autoregulatory range of perfusion pressures (90–200mmHg), blood flow is independent of perfusion pressure so, as the perfusion pressure increases,

Fig. 3.4 Autoregulation of glomerular filtration rate (GFR) and renal blood flow (RBF).

resistance to flow increases (Fig. 3.4). Two mechanisms are involved in autoregulation:
1. Myogenic mechanism.
2. Tubuloglomerular feedback mechanism.

Myogenic mechanism

An increase in pressure (caused by an increase in blood flow) stimulates stretch receptors in smooth muscle fibres in the vessel wall. This causes reflex contraction of smooth muscle fibres, resulting in vessel vasoconstriction. There is an increased resistance to flow so, overall, RBF remains constant.

Tubuloglomerular feedback mechanism

This monitors the NaCl concentration at the macula densa (which detects pressure/flow changes within the kidney). Changes in the pressure/flow are transmitted from the macula densa to cells in the juxtaglomerular apparatus (JGA), which produce vasoactive substances to counteract the changes and therefore cause the GFR to return to normal. For example, if GFR rises, the tubular flow rate also increases, so fewer Na^+ and Cl^- are reabsorbed and a higher concentration is detected at the macula densa. This stimulates the JGA to release vasoconstrictor substances. The main mediator involved in this mechanism is angiotensin II and, to a lesser extent, prostaglandins and adenosine.

Renal blood flow and systemic blood pressure

Autoregulation maintains a constant blood flow to the kidneys despite changes in blood pressure. However, the blood flow itself is not always constant, for example, acute haemorrhage results in increased sympathetic activity to the kidney (and other parts of the body). This leads to vasoconstriction and consequently a decreased blood flow. Intrarenal vasodilator prostaglandins are produced to prevent excessive vasoconstriction and renal perfusion is thus maintained.

Regulation of GFR involves other vasoactive substances, which are found in the walls of blood vessels. These are summarized in Fig. 3.5.

Age-related changes in RBF and GFR

Age-related changes in RBF and GFR (Fig. 3.6) are as follows:

- Week 10 of gestation (in utero): filtration of fluid and urine production begin; this contributes to the amniotic fluid.
- Newborn: GFR $\approx 25\,mL/min/1.73\,m^2$ body surface area. RBF $\approx 5\%$ of cardiac output—this increases progressively during the first year.

- 1 month old: progressive increase in GFR (PAH cannot be used to measure RBF because tubular secretion is not developed, so extraction of PAH is less than 100%).
- By 1 year of age: GFR reaches adult values (120 mL/min).
- Adults: RBF $\approx 20\%$ of cardiac output.
- Old age: GFR decreases progressively.

Body fluid osmolality

Concepts of osmolality

Body weight remains relatively constant from day to day because total body water remains constant. The normal intake and output of water are discussed in Chapter 1. At least 400 mL/day of urine must be produced for the kidney to maintain homeostasis.

The normal plasma osmolality (P_{osm}) is 285–295 mOsmol/kgH$_2$O. This is strictly regulated and an increase or decrease of 3 mOsmol/kgH$_2$O will stimulate the body's osmolality regulation mechanism.

Vasoactive substances found in the blood vessel walls	
Vasodilator	**Vasoconstrictor**
prostaglandins (PGs)	adenosine
nitric oxide (NO)	angiotensin II
dopamine (DA)	antidiuretic hormone (ADH)
bradykinin	endothelin
	norepinephrine (NE)

Fig. 3.5 Vasoactive substances found in the blood vessel walls.

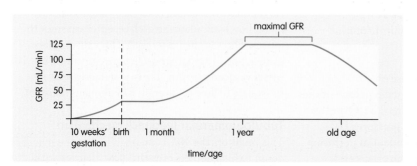

Fig. 3.6 Age-related changes in glomerular filtration rate (GFR).

Fig. 3.7 Role of antidiuretic hormone (ADH) in maintaining osmolality. ECF, extracellular fluid.

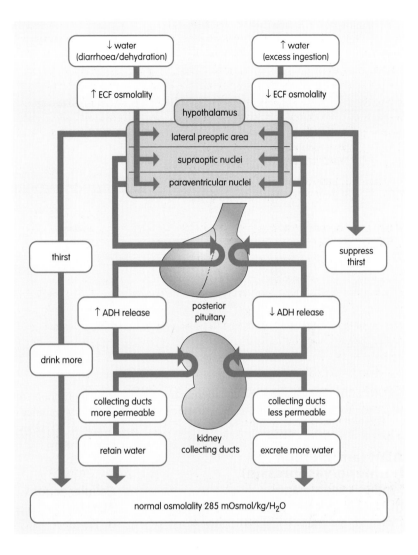

Total body water balance depends upon:
- Regulation of water excretion by the kidneys.
- Water intake via the thirst mechanism.

Both are controlled by the osmoreceptors.

Osmoreceptors

Osmoreceptors detect changes in the plasma osmolality and are located in the supraoptic and paraventricular areas of the anterior hypothalamus. Their blood supply is the internal carotid artery. They have two functions:

1. To regulate the release of antidiuretic hormone (ADH, also known as vasopressin).
2. To regulate thirst (this also depends on other osmoreceptors in the lateral preoptic area of the hypothalamus).

Figure 3.7 illustrates the role of ADH in maintaining osmolality.

Sensitivity of osmoreceptors to osmotic changes caused by different solutes

Na^+ and other associated anions are the main constituents that determine plasma osmolality. Water loss alters the Na^+ concentration. Other solutes without the addition or loss of water can also change the osmolality. Not all solutes stimulate the osmoreceptors to the same degree—this depends

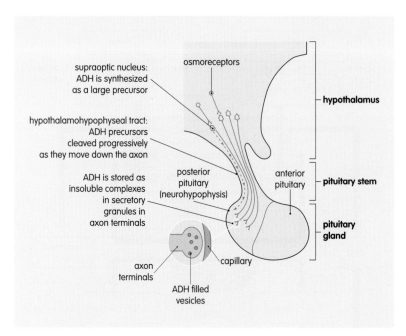

Fig. 3.8 Synthesis and storage of antidiuretic hormone (ADH).

supraoptic nucleus: ADH is synthesized as a large precursor

osmoreceptors

hypothalamus

hypothalamohypophyseal tract: ADH precursors cleaved progressively as they move down the axon

ADH is stored as insoluble complexes in secretory granules in axon terminals

posterior pituitary (neurohypophysis)

anterior pituitary

pituitary stem

pituitary gland

axon terminals

capillary

ADH filled vesicles

on how easily they can cross the cell membrane (i.e. their ability to cause cellular dehydration).

ADH (antidiuretic hormone/vasopressin)
Synthesis and storage
ADH is a peptide hormone synthesized in the supraoptic nucleus of the hypothalamus as a large precursor molecule. It is transported to the posterior pituitary gland, where its synthesis is completed and it is stored until release (Fig. 3.8).

Release
A rise in plasma osmolality triggers ADH release. Action potentials in the neurons from the hypothalamus (which contains ADH) depolarize the axon membrane, resulting in Ca^{2+} influx, fusion of secretory granules with the axon membrane and the release of ADH and neurophysin into the bloodstream.

Cellular actions
ADH has two functions:
1. To reduce water excretion (V_2 receptor mediated).
2. To stimulate blood vessel vasoconstriction (V_1 receptor mediated).

When present on the peritubular side of the collecting tubule cell (Fig. 3.9), ADH causes intracellular water channels (aquaporins) to fuse with the luminal membrane. ADH is not effective if present on the luminal side of the tubule because

 ADH secretion is controlled by:
- Osmoreceptors (which detect changes in the body fluid osmolarity).
- Baroreceptors (which detect changes in blood volume, i.e. blood vessel wall 'stretch').

The osmoreceptor system is more sensitive than the baroreceptor system.

Fig. 3.9 Actions of antidiuretic hormone (ADH) in the collecting tubule. AC, adenylate cyclase; cAMP, cyclic adenosine monophosphate; PKA, protein kinase.

there are no ADH receptors (V_2 receptors) on the basal membrane of the tubular cells. The V_2 receptors are G-protein-coupled receptors, which have a seven membrane-spanning region. The relationship between urine osmolality (mOsmol/kg) and plasma ADH concentration is shown in Fig. 3.10.

Fate of ADH
ADH must be removed rapidly from the blood once plasma osmolarity has been corrected. This is done by the liver and kidneys (50%), with less than 10% appearing in the urine; the rest is metabolized. Its short plasma half-life (10–15min) also ensures that the duration of its effect in the blood is limited.

Drugs affecting ADH release
Drugs can:
- Increase ADH release (e.g. nicotine, ether, morphine, barbiturates).
- Inhibit ADH release (e.g. alcohol).

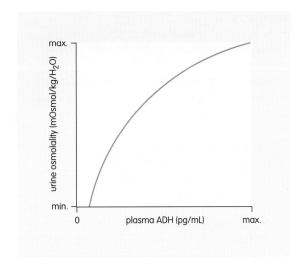

Fig. 3.10 Urine osmolality in relation to plasma antidiuretic hormone (ADH) concentration (from Berne RM, Levy MN 1996 Physiology, 3rd edn. Mosby Year Book).

Causes of SIADH	
Disorder	**Example of finding**
CNS disorders	abscess, stroke, vasculitis (systemic lupus erythematosus)
malignancy	small cell carcinoma in lungs, duodenum, pancreas, prostate, ureter, adrenals
lung diseases	tuberculosis, pneumonia, abscess, aspergillosis
drugs	opiates, chlorpropamide, psychotropics, cytotoxics, narcotics, oxytocin
metabolic diseases	porphyria, hypothyroidism
miscellaneous	pain (postoperative), Guillain–Barré syndrome, trauma

Fig. 3.11 Causes of syndrome of inappropriate antidiuretic hormone secretion (SIADH).

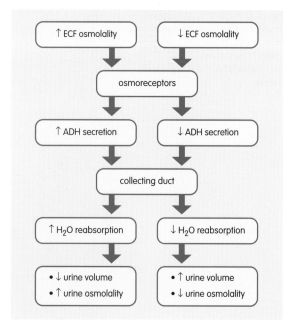

Fig. 3.12 Summary of antidiuretic hormone (ADH) action. ECF, extracellular fluid.

Syndrome of inappropriate ADH (SIADH) secretion

Occasionally ADH is secreted inappropriately by the pituitary or other areas in the body. Causes are given in Fig. 3.11. Signs and symptoms are:
- Hyponatraemia (<125mmol/L) and low plasma osmolality (<260mmol/L).
- Inappropriate urine osmolality: the urine concentration is higher than normal (i.e. not maximally diluted).
- Inappropriate Na^+ excretion: urinary $[Na^+]$ is greater than 20mmol/L despite a decrease in plasma Na^+ concentration because the plasma volume is maintained by water retention (unless volume contracted or sodium restricted, which can decrease urinary Na^+).

The diagnosis should be considered in hyponatraemic patients in the absence of hypovolemia, oedema, endocrine dysfunction, renal failure and drugs, all of which can impair water excretion.

Diabetes insipidus

This is the inability to reabsorb water from the distal part of the nephron, due to the failure of secretion or action of ADH. Symptoms are:
- Polyuria.
- Polydipsia.
- Low urine osmolality, i.e. dilute urine.

The causes of diabetes insipidus are:
- Neurogenic/central: impaired ADH synthesis or secretion by the hypothalamus, which might be congenital, caused by hypothalamic damage or due to pituitary tumours. It can be treated by administering ADH.
- Nephrogenic: failure of the kidneys to respond to circulating ADH, which could be caused by mutations in the gene coding for V_2 receptors, chronic pyelonephritis, polycystic kidneys or drugs such as lithium. Plasma ADH levels are normal. There is no current treatment to correct the deficit.

Diabetes insipidus can be mistaken for psychogenic polydipsia, where large volumes of dilute urine are produced secondary to compulsive water drinking. This causes a decrease in the urine-concentrating ability because of loss of medullary tonicity.

Figure 3.12 summarizes the action of ADH.

Water clearance and reabsorption

Dehydration leads to a rise in plasma osmolality. Thus, the kidneys reabsorb 'solute-free' water from the tubules. This produces a more dilute plasma and a concentrated urine.

Fig. 3.13 Osmotic clearance.

$$C_{osm} = \frac{U_{osm} \times V}{P_{osm}}$$

If urine is isotonic then $\frac{U_{osm}}{P_{osm}} = 1$ $\therefore C_{osm} = V$

Key

U_{osm}	=	urine osmolality
P_{osm}	=	plasma osmolality
V	=	volume
C_{osm}	=	osmotic clearance
C_{H_2O}	=	free water clearance
T_{CH_2O}	=	free water reabsorption

If urine osmolality < plasma osmolality, i.e. dilute urine production:

$$\frac{U_{osm}}{P_{osm}} < 1 \quad \therefore C_{osm} < V$$

The urine volume has additional free water and isotonic fluid

$$\therefore V = C_{osm} + C_{H_2O}$$

Maximum C_{H_2O} = 12–15 mL/min (15–22 L/day)

If urine osmolality > plasma osmolality, i.e. concentrated urine produced:

$$\frac{U_{osm}}{P_{osm}} > 1 \quad \therefore C_{osm} > V$$

Here however, water is being excreted so

$$\therefore V = C_{osm} - T_{CH_2O}$$

Water is reabsorbed here so we can substitute (C_{H_2O}) for T_{CH_2O}

C_{H_2O} and T_{CH_2O} are quantitative ways of determining the ability of the kidney to excrete or conserve water

Excessive water intake lowers plasma osmolality. Thus, the kidneys excrete 'solute-free' water from the tubules, producing dilute urine. Dilute urine has a lower osmolality than plasma, concentrated urine has a higher osmolality than plasma, isotonic urine has the same osmolality as plasma. The osmotic clearance (C_{osm} Fig. 3.13) is the rate at which osmotically active substances are cleared from the plasma. If urine is isotonic, C_{osm} = urine flow (Fig. 3.13).

Effect of solute output on urine volume

The concentrating ability of the kidneys is limited, with a maximum urinary osmolality of 1400 mOsmol/kg. Thus, the amount of urine excreted per day depends on the:

- Amount of ADH.
- Amount of solute excreted.

At maximum ADH concentration, large amounts of solutes can still cause a diuresis (see Fig. 3.14).

Mannitol is an osmotic diuretic that cannot be reabsorbed. It alters the kidney's concentrating ability and produces isotonic urine. In diabetes

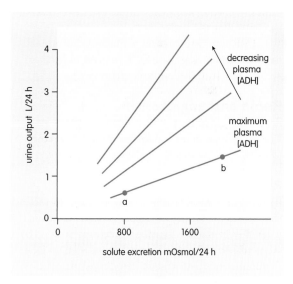

Fig. 3.14 Effect of antidiuretic hormone (ADH) on urine output. a, minimum possible urine output with a solute excretion of 800mOsmol/24h; b, minimum urine output if 2000mOsmol/24h must be excreted.

47

mellitus, the excess blood glucose causes an osmotic diuresis.

Adrenal steroids and urinary dilution

Adrenal insufficiency leads to impaired water excretion (i.e. mineralocorticoid and/or glucocorticoid deficiency):

- Glucocorticoid deficiency can enhance water permeability of the collecting duct.
- Glucocorticoid and mineralocorticoid deficiencies increase ADH levels, resulting in an inability to produce dilute urine. This is corrected by administering adrenal steroids.

Body fluid volume

Basic concepts
Effective circulating volume

The volume of fluid that perfuses tissues is the effective circulating volume; this needs to be kept constant. Na^+ is the major extracellular ion and affects the ECF volume, for example, a rise in ECF Na^+ results in increased osmolality, which leads to water retention and thirst (increased drinking of water). This increases ECF volume and normalizes osmolality. Thus, the ECF volume can be regulated by controlling the body's Na^+.

If ECF volume decreases sufficiently, intrarenal mechanisms can decrease GFR to prevent further volume loss (tubuloglomerular feedback).

Renin and angiotensin
Renin–angiotensin–aldosterone system

The renin–angiotensin–aldosterone (RAA) system (Fig. 3.15) maintains Na^+ balance.

Renin

Renin is an enzyme that is synthesized and stored in the JGA in the kidneys. A fall in plasma Na^+ leads to a fall in ECF volume, causing the release of renin by:

- Increased sympathetic innervation: a fall in ECF volume results in a fall in blood pressure. This is detected by baroreceptors in carotid arteries and causes increased sympathetic activity. Granular cells of the JGA are innervated by the sympathetic system, so an increase in sympathetic activity leads to an increase in renin release. The process is mediated by β-adrenergic receptors.
- The wall tension in afferent arterioles falls: decreased ECF volume reduces blood pressure,

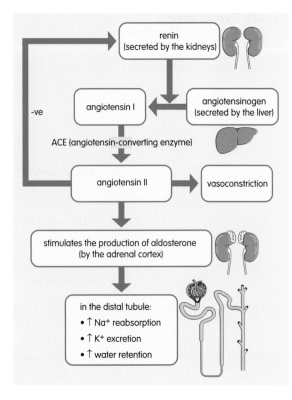

Fig. 3.15 The renin–angiotensin–aldosterone system. –ve, negative feedback.

which in turn decreases perfusion pressure to the kidneys. Changes in the blood pressure decrease wall tension at granular cells, which stimulates renin release.

- Decreased Na^+ to the macula densa: if less NaCl reaches the macula densa, the macula densa is stimulated to secrete the prostaglandin PGI_2. This acts on the granular cells to cause renin release.

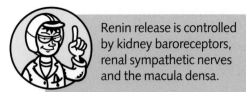

Renin release is controlled by kidney baroreceptors, renal sympathetic nerves and the macula densa.

Conversion of angiotensinogen to angiotensin

Renin acts on angiotensinogen (α_2-globulin), which splits off angiotensin I (a decapeptide). Angiotensin converting enzyme (ACE) in the lungs then removes two amino acids to produce angiotensin II (an octapeptide). Angiotensin II:

- Stimulates the zona glomerulosa of the adrenal cortex to release aldosterone.

Fig. 3.16 Factors causing aldosterone release and the effects of aldosterone. ECF, extracellular fluid.

- Directly vasoconstricts arterioles within the kidney (efferent > afferent).
- Directly increases Na^+ reabsorption from the proximal tubule.
- Releases ADH.
- Stimulates thirst.
- Provides negative feedback to the JGA cells, and therefore affects renin release (Fig. 3.15).

In addition to the generation of circulating angiotensin II, the local generation of angiotensin II by ACE (within the tissues) might have an important pathogenic role. ACE inhibitors are used to treat high blood pressure. They decrease the production of angiotensin II and consequently:
- Decrease vasoconstriction.
- Decrease aldosterone (and prevent an increase in ECF volume).

Aldosterone

Aldosterone is synthesized by zona glomerulosa cells in the adrenal cortex. Its release (Fig. 3.16) is controlled by:
- Angiotensin II.
- ECF volume: if circulating Na^+ falls, effective circulating volume also falls. This stimulates aldosterone release via the renin–angiotensin–aldosterone system.
- Na^+ concentration: via direct aldosterone release from the adrenal cortex, as well as through the renin–angiotensin–aldosterone system.
- K^+ concentration: a rise in circulating K^+ stimulates direct release of aldosterone from the

adrenal cortex. This returns K^+ to normal by increasing distal tubular secretion of K^+.

Aldosterone primarily regulates sodium concentration. It acts within cells to:
- Promote Na^+ reabsorption in the kidney, colon, gastric glands and sweat and salivary gland ducts.
- Promote K^+ and H^+ secretion by the kidney.

Factors affecting Na⁺ reabsorption
Starling forces in the proximal tubule
The amount of Na^+ and water reabsorbed into the peritubular capillaries from the proximal tubule depends on the rate and amount of uptake from the lateral intercellular spaces into the capillaries.

Changes in the body fluid volume alters plasma hydrostatic and oncotic pressure, for example, increased NaCl intake is mirrored by a rise in ECF volume. This in turn increases hydrostatic pressure and decreases oncotic pressure, so NaCl and water reabsorption by the proximal tubule cells decreases.

Sympathetic drive from the renal nerves
The arterial baroreceptors regulate renal sympathetic nerve activity, for example, a fall in ECF volume decreases blood pressure, which is sensed by baroreceptors, and results in an increase in sympathetic activity. This stimulates Na^+ retention and an increase in peripheral resistance, thus restoring ECF volume and blood pressure.

A rise in sympathetic nerve activity to the kidney stimulates renin release either directly or as a result of renal vasoconstriction (this activates the JGA). Catecholamines from sympathetic nerve endings also stimulate Na^+ reabsorption by the proximal tubule, but it is unclear if this is a direct effect or secondary to altered peritubular forces.

Prostaglandins

A decrease in the effective circulating volume stimulates cortical prostaglandin (PG) synthesis. In the kidney, PG synthesis occurs in the:
- Cortex (arterioles and glomeruli).
- Medullary interstitial cells.
- Collecting duct epithelial cells.

Several prostaglandins exist: PGE_2 (medullary), PGI_2 (cortical), $PGF_2\alpha$, PGD_2 and TXA_2 (thromboxane). The main functions of each are as follows:
- PGE_2, PGI_2: vasodilators, preventing excessive vasoconstriction.
- PGI_2 (prostacyclin): renin release.
- PGE_2 (medullary): promotes water (diuretic) and sodium (natriuretic) excretion within the collecting tubules and thus overrides the antidiuretic action of ADH. PGE_2 protects the medullary tubule cells from excessive hypoxia when the ECF volume decreases.
- TXA_2: a vasoconstrictor, which is synthesized after repeated kidney damage (e.g. ureteral obstruction). It reduces the amount of blood available for filtration by a poorly functioning kidney.

Atrial natriuretic peptide (ANP)

ANP is a peptide produced by cardiac atrial cells in response to an increase in ECF volume. It is found in the atrial cells and released into the plasma. ANP binds to specific cell surface receptors, resulting in increased cyclic guanosine monosulphate (cGMP). ANP acts to:
- Inhibit Na^+/K^+ ATPase and close Na^+ channels of the collecting ducts, reducing Na^+ reabsorption. Na^+ reabsorption is also reduced in the proximal tubules. Thus, Na^+ and water excretion by the kidney is increased.
- Vasodilate afferent arterioles, thereby increasing GFR.
- Inhibit aldosterone secretion.
- Inhibit ADH release.
- Decrease renin release.

Dopamine

This is synthesized by the proximal tubule cells and:
- Inhibits Na^+/K^+ ATPase and Na^+/H^+ antiport, thereby decreasing tubular Na^+ transport.
- Increases Na^+ excretion (natriuresis).
- Causes vasodilation.

Kinins

Kininogens are cleaved by the enzyme kallikrein to form kinins. The effects of kinins are similar to PGs and include:
- Vasodilation.
- Inhibition of ADH release.
- Increased Na^+ excretion.

Natriuretic hormone

This hormone inhibits the Na^+/K^+ ATPase enzyme and is thought to be produced by the hypothalamus.

Figure 3.17 summarizes the mechanisms involved in the regulation of body fluid.

Regulation of body fluid pH

Body fluid pH is tightly controlled because most enzyme reactions are sensitive to pH changes.
- Normal pH range is 7.35–7.45.
- Normal H^+ concentration is 35–45 nmol/L.

Buffers
Definition

A buffer is a mixture of a weak acid (HA) and a conjugate base. It undergoes minimal pH change when either an acid or a base is added to it:

$$HA \leftrightarrow H^+ \text{ (acid)} + A^- \text{ (conjugate base)}$$

It can also be a mixture of a weak base (BH) and conjugate acid:

$$BH \leftrightarrow H^+ \text{ (conjugate acid)} + B^- \text{ (base)}$$

For example, if there is an increase in H^+, the equations above shift to the left so that the extra H^+ combines with the buffer and the H^+ concentration in the body falls.

The kidneys act together with the lungs and buffer systems to minimize any changes in plasma $[H^+]$.

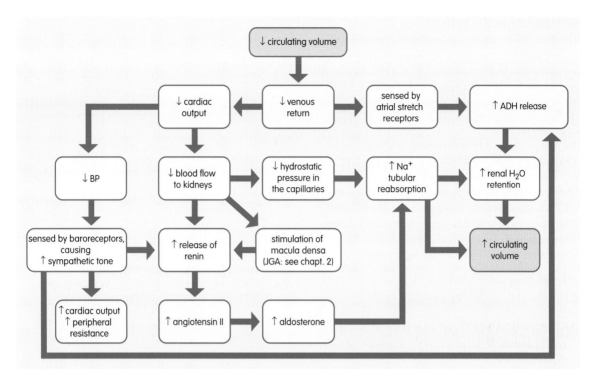

Fig. 3.17 Regulation of body fluid. JGA, juxtaglomerular apparatus.

pK values and equilibrium constants

The equations below demonstrate the equilibrium constants in terms of conjugate acids and bases, proton donators, and acceptors.

$$HA \leftrightarrow H^+ + A^-$$

Equation 1. At equilibrium:

$$K = \frac{[H^+][A^-]}{[HA]}$$

$$\therefore [H^+] = \frac{K[HA]}{[A^-]}$$

$$= \frac{K[acid]}{[base]}$$

Equation 2:

$$pH = -\log[H^+]$$

$$= \frac{\log 1}{[H^+]}$$

$$pK = -\log K$$

$$= \frac{\log 1}{K}$$

Equation 3. Combining equations 1 and 2 (the Henderson–Hasselbalch equation).

Buffer systems in different body compartments

Buffer systems	Blood	ECF and CSF	ICF
HCO_3^-/CO_2	×	×	×
haemoglobin	×		
plasma proteins	×		
phosphate	×	×	×
organic phosphate			×
proteins		×	×

Fig. 3.18 Buffer systems in different body compartments. CSF, cerebrospinal fluid; ECF, extracellular fluid; ICF, intracellular fluid.

$$pH = \frac{pK + \log[base]}{[acid]}$$

Physiological buffers

There are several buffer systems in the different body compartments (Fig. 3.18), of which the most important is the bicarbonate buffer system.

Bicarbonate buffer system

The bicarbonate buffer system is important in all body fluids. Carbon dioxide (CO_2) and water (H_2O) are combined to form carbonic acid (H_2CO_3) by the enzyme carbonic anhydrase (CA). The H_2CO_3 then dissociates spontaneously to form bicarbonate ions (HCO_3^-) and H^+. This is summarized in the equation below:

$$CO_2 + H_2O \xrightleftharpoons{\text{Carbonic anhydrase}} H_2CO_3 \leftrightarrow H^+ + HCO_3^-$$

CO_2 concentration is regulated by the lungs and HCO_3^- concentration is regulated by the kidneys. Therefore, pH regulation depends equally on both these organs. Substituting this equation in the Henderson–Hasselbalch equation, we get:

$$pH = pK + \log [HCO_3^-]/[H_2CO_3]$$

$[H_2CO_3]$ is determined by dissolved CO_2:

$[H_2CO_3] = 0.23 \times pCO_2$ (0.23 is the CO_2 solubility coefficient at 37°C; pCO_2 is the pressure of CO_2 in the lungs)

Therefore, $pH = pK + \log[HCO_3^-]/0.23 \times pCO_2$
    Normal values are:
- $[HCO_3^-]$: 20–30mmol/L.
- pCO_2: 4.4–5.3kPa.
- pK of HCO_3^-/pCO_2 system: 6.1.

Therefore pH = 7.4. In summary:

$$pH \propto HCO_3^-/pCO_2$$

Renal regulation of plasma HCO_3^-

H^+ is produced during metabolism, which stimulates CO_2 production:

$$H^+ + HCO_3^- \leftrightarrow H_2CO_3 \leftrightarrow H_2O + CO_2$$

CO_2 is exhaled by the lungs. The kidneys retain HCO_3^- and make more HCO_3^-.

The concentration of HCO_3^- in the plasma filtered by the kidney is 25mmol/L. HCO_3^- is reabsorbed by the kidney using a T_m-dependent mechanism (Fig. 3.19). The T_m is similar to the amount of HCO_3^- filtered at a normal plasma concentration. If plasma HCO_3^- increases, T_m is exceeded and HCO_3^- is excreted until the plasma level returns to normal. Figure 3.19 illustrates the way in which HCO_3^- is handled by the kidney.

Ninety per cent of HCO_3^- is absorbed in the proximal tubule (see Chapter 2).

Fig. 3.19 How HCO_3^- ions are handled by the kidney. HCO_3^- absorption is dependent on H^+ secretion into the tubule. This dependency causes the T_m for HCO_3^- absorption to vary. The limits of the T_m variability are illustrated by the dotted lines on the graph above.

HCO_3^- reabsorption

In the proximal tubule: the lumen

HCO_3^- reacts with H^+ (delivered into the lumen via an antiport process coupled with Na^+) to give H_2CO_3. H_2CO_3 dissociates into H_2O and CO_2, catalysed by the enzyme CA (present in the brush border of luminal cells). CA inhibitors suppress H^+ secretion, leading to a fall in Na^+ and HCO_3^- absorption, and thus act as a weak diuretic.

In the proximal tubule: the tubular cells

H_2O and CO_2 enter the tubular cells and reform H_2CO_3, catalysed by CA. H_2CO_3 again dissociates into:
- H^+, which is secreted into the lumen.
- HCO_3^-, which enters the plasma via the peritubular fluid (see also Chapter 2).

Some HCO_3^- couples with luminal Cl^- so that HCO_3^- is secreted into the lumen and Cl^- is absorbed.

In the distal tubule

This involves intercalated cells. Secreted H^+ and luminal HCO_3^- are present but CA is limited. Therefore little CO_2 and H_2O are produced, so less HCO_3^- is absorbed. H^+ ions are secreted across into the lumen by H^+ ATPase and H^+/K^+ ATPase (pumps H^+ out and K^+ in).

Fig. 3.20 Conversion of alkaline phosphate to acid phosphate in the tubule lumen. This conversion liberates free sodium, which is transported into the tubule cell by an Na^+/H^+ antiporter, causing H^+ secretion into the lumen and increased HCO_3^- reabsorption by the tubule cells. CA, carbonic anhydrase.

Conversion of alkaline phosphate to acid phosphate—luminal buffer

Alkaline phosphate Na_2HPO_4 and acid phosphate NaH_2PO_4 are present in the plasma in the ratio of 4:1. Both are filtered at the glomerulus. Alkaline phosphate is converted to acid phosphate, mainly in the distal tubule but also in the proximal tubule (Fig. 3.20). This generates HCO_3^- for the plasma.

Ammonia secretion—luminal buffer

Deamination of glutamine in the proximal tubule produces ammonium ions (NH_4^+) (see Fig. 3.20). Although the liver can metabolize NH_4^+ to urea, it is only by secretion of NH_4^+ in the kidney that HCO_3^- can be regenerated to act as a buffer in the plasma. However, 50% of NH_4^+ secreted into the proximal tubule is reabsorbed by the thick ascending limb of the loop of Henle and accumulates in the cells of the medullary interstitium (see Fig. 3.22). Figure 3.21

illustrates the secretion and handling of ammonia (NH_3) and Fig. 3.22 shows NH_3 and NH_4^+ handling by the nephrons.

Acidosis increases NH_4^+ excretion because:
- Acidosis stimulates enzymes that deaminate glutamine, thereby increasing NH_4^+ synthesis.
- Increased H^+ secretion results in NH_3 production, which in turn results in increased NH_4^+ in the collecting tubules. The conversion of NH_3 to NH_4^+ maintains a gradient for NH_3 secretion. In this way, excess NH_3/NH_4^+ is removed from the medulla.

Acid–base disturbances

There are four main types:
1. Respiratory acidosis.
2. Respiratory alkalosis.
3. Metabolic (non-respiratory origin) acidosis.
4. Metabolic alkalosis.

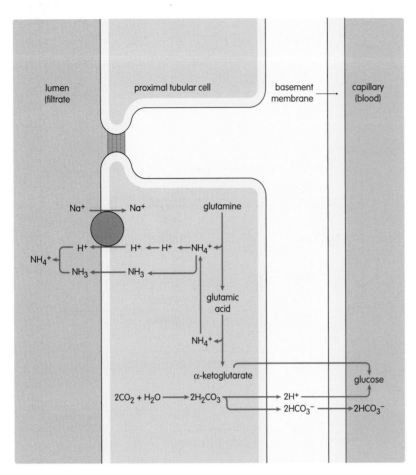

Fig. 3.21 Renal secretion and handling of NH_3.

Metabolic disturbances result from changes in cellular metabolism or diet, so are independent of pCO_2 changes. If the body fluid pH alters, the buffering system mechanism is activated. Thus, overall, there might be very little change in arterial pH despite acid–base imbalance. A change in the arterial pH results in a change in the pH of body cells, which adversely affects many cellular processes.

The Davenport diagram is a graph of the plasma HCO_3^- versus plasma pH, used to classify acid–base disturbances (Fig. 3.23).

Compensation and correction
- Compensation is the restoration of normal pH even when acid–base imbalance is still present.
- Correction is the restoration of both the pH and acid–base imbalance to normal:

$$H_2O + CO_2 \leftrightarrow H_2CO_3 \leftrightarrow H^+ + HCO_3^-$$

$$pH \propto [HCO_3^-]/pCO_2$$

Therefore, if two variables (e.g. pH and pCO_2) are known, $[HCO_3^-]$ can be calculated.

Arterial blood gases (ABG) measure the pH, pO_2 and pCO_2 in an arterial blood sample. This can be used to diagnose an acid–base imbalance. For example, if pH = 7.2 and pCO_2 is 9.3 kPa, by looking at Fig. 3.23 it can be seen that $[HCO_3^-]$ will be raised. This corresponds to a respiratory acidosis.

Examples of acid–base disturbances
Respiratory acidosis
The causes of respiratory acidosis are:
- Chronic bronchitis.
- Emphysema.
- Obstruction of the airway (e.g. tumour, foreign body).
- Mechanical chest injuries.
- Severe asthma.
- Drugs: general anaesthetic, morphine, barbiturates (respiratory centre depressant).
- Injuries and infections to the respiratory centre in the brainstem.

Fig. 3.22 Handling of NH_3 and NH_4^+ by nephrons.

Fig. 3.23 Acid and base disturbances with compensatory changes demonstrated on the Davenport diagram.

ABG results show $pCO_2 > 6.0\,kPa$ and decreased pH. Clinically, the respiratory system cannot remove enough CO_2, so CO_2 increases together with pCO_2. Therefore the following equation is shifted to the right:

$$\overrightarrow{CO_2 + H_2O} \leftrightarrow H_2CO_3 \leftrightarrow H^+ + HCO_3^-$$

This results in elevated $[H^+]$ and $[HCO_3^-]$. The extra H^+ results in increased H^+ secretion and increased HCO_3^- reabsorption. This restores pH, acting as a compensatory response. The acid–base disturbance is not corrected because the pCO_2 and $[HCO_3^-]$ are still high. Correction requires hyperventilation to decrease pCO_2.

Figure 3.23 illustrates acid–base disturbances with compensatory changes.

Respiratory alkalosis

The causes of respiratory alkalosis are:

- Decreased pO_2, which is detected by chemoreceptors in the carotid body, resulting in hyperventilation and decreased pCO_2.
- High altitude.
- Fever.
- Brainstem damage resulting in hyperventilation.
- Hysterical overbreathing.

The ABG results show a $pCO_2 < 4.7\,kPa$ and an elevated pH. Clinically, too much CO_2 is removed by the respiratory system. Therefore the following equation is shifted to the left:

$$\overleftarrow{CO_2 + H_2O} \leftrightarrow H_2CO_3 \leftrightarrow H^+ + HCO_3^-$$

This causes $[H^+]$ to fall and hence an increased pH and a slight decrease in $[HCO_3^-]$. The compensatory response involves reduced H^+ secretion, increased HCO_3^- excretion and decreased HCO_3^- reabsorption, thus restoring pH. Correction involves rectification of the underlying respiratory defect.

Metabolic acidosis

The causes of metabolic acidosis are:

- Ingestion of acids (H^+).
- Excess metabolic production of H^+ (e.g. lactate acidosis, diabetic ketoacidosis).
- Loss of HCO_3^- (e.g. severe diarrhoea, drainage from fistulae).
- Renal disease (failure to excrete H^+).

ABG results show a normal pCO_2 and decreased pH. There is an increase in $[H^+]$. Therefore, the following equation is shifted to the left:

$$\overleftarrow{CO_2 + H_2O} \leftrightarrow H_2CO_3 \leftrightarrow H^+ + HCO_3^-$$

Consequently, $[HCO_3^-]$ falls as it is used to 'mop up' the excess H^+ ions.

The decreased pH stimulates respiration to cause hyperventilation. This respiratory compensation decreases pCO_2 and returns the pH to normal, although HCO_3^- falls further. The fall in HCO_3^- hinders the compensatory response of the kidneys, which is to increase HCO_3^- reabsorption and produce titratable acid.

The anion gap represents the difference between plasma anions and cations and represents unaccounted anions (e.g. phosphates, ketones, lactate):

$$\text{Anion gap} = ([K^+] + [Na^+]) - ([Cl^-] + [HCO_3^-])$$

The normal range is 8–16 mmol/L. Changes in the anion gap help define the cause of a metabolic acidosis. Metabolic acidosis due to diarrhoea or renal tubular acidosis does not alter the anion gap. Acidosis caused by renal failure, diabetes or lactic acidosis increases the anion gap.

Metabolic alkalosis

The causes of metabolic alkalosis are:

- Loss of acid (e.g. vomiting, diarrhoea).
- Ingestion of alkali (e.g. antacid ingestion)
- Depleted ECF (e.g. haemorrhage, burns, excess diuretic use, contraction alkalosis).

ABG results show a normal pCO_2 and an elevated pH because of a rise in plasma $[HCO_3^-]$. Therefore, the following equation is shifted to the right:

$$\overrightarrow{CO_2 + H_2O} \leftrightarrow H_2CO_3 \leftrightarrow H^+ + HCO_3^-$$
$$H^+ + OH^- \to H_2O$$

Consequently, $[HCO_3^-]$ is increased.

Respiratory compensation occurs. The increase in pH acts on chemoreceptors, which reduce the ventilatory rate and so increase pCO_2. The equation therefore shifts to the right and the pH returns to normal, but HCO_3^- increases further. This hinders correction (see Fig. 3.23).

Figure 3.24 summarizes acid–base disturbances.

Regulation of calcium and phosphate

Calcium (Ca²⁺)

Ca^{2+} is present mainly in bone but has an important extraskeletal function. The threshold potential of

Fig. 3.24 Summary of acid–base disturbances and compensatory mechanisms.

Summary of acid–base disturbances and compensatory mechanisms					
Acid–base disturbance	pH	pCO_2	HCO_3^-	Clinical cause	Compensation
respiratory acidosis	↓	↑	↑	severe asthma; COPD	metabolic (↑ HCO_3^-)
respiratory alkalosis	↑	↓	↓	hyperventilation	metabolic (↑ HCO_3^-)
metabolic acidosis	↓	normal	↓	diabetic ketoacidosis; chronic renal failure	respiratory (↓ pCO_2)
metabolic alkalosis	↑	normal	↑	vomiting	respiratory (↓ pCO_2)

cell membranes of nerve and muscle for action potentials varies inversely with plasma calcium concentration. Thus it is important to keep calcium levels constant.

Calcium exists in two forms in the plasma:

1. Ionized Ca^{2+}, which is physiologically more important (normal concentration: 1.25 mmol/L).
2. Ca^{2+} bound to protein—mainly albumin (normal concentration: 1.25 mmol/L).

Ca^{2+} concentrations are:

- Total plasma Ca^{2+}: 2.2–2.6 mmol/L.
- ECF Ca^{2+}: 1.25 mmol/L.
- Interstitial fluid total Ca^{2+}: 1.25 mmol/L.
- Intracellular Ca^{2+}: 0.0001 mmol/L; found in smooth endothelial reticulum and mitochondria, complexed with calmodulin.

It is important to maintain a low intracellular Ca^{2+}.

Clinical features and causes of Ca^{2+} disturbances

Hypocalcaemia

Causes are:

- Hypoparathyroidism.
- Rickets and osteomalacia (low vitamin D).
- Hypomagnesaemia.
- Pancreatitis.
- Alkalosis, which reduces the amount of H^+ available to bind to protein, so more Ca^{2+} can bind to protein. This results in decreased ionized Ca^{2+}, although total Ca^{2+} remains the same.
- Chronic renal failure, due to hyperphosphataemia (if PO_4^{3-} rises, Ca^{2+} must fall proportionally) and low levels of activated vitamin D.

Decreased Ca^{2+} results in tetany with convulsions, hand and feet muscle cramps (leading to paralysis) and cardiac arrhythmias.

Hypercalcaemia

Causes of hypercalcaemia are:

- Primary hyperparathyroidism.
- Sudden acidosis, resulting in the release of bound calcium, which becomes ionized Ca^{2+}.
- Increased intestinal absorption due to excess vitamin D or ingestion of calcium (milk–alkali syndrome).
- Bone destruction resulting in increased Ca^{2+} release from bone—usually caused by secondary deposits from malignancy or myeloma.
- Production of humoral hypercalcaemic agents by tumours.
- Granulomatous disease (sarcoid).
- Drugs, e.g. thiazides.
- Tertiary hyperparathyroidism in chronic renal failure.
- Hypermagnesaemia.

Symptoms of hypercalcaemia are:

- Renal calculi.
- Behaviour disturbance (because of the effects on higher cerebral functions).
- Constipation due to decreased intestinal mobility.
- Renal damage.
- Calcification outside the skeletal system.
- Polyuria.
- Polydipsia.

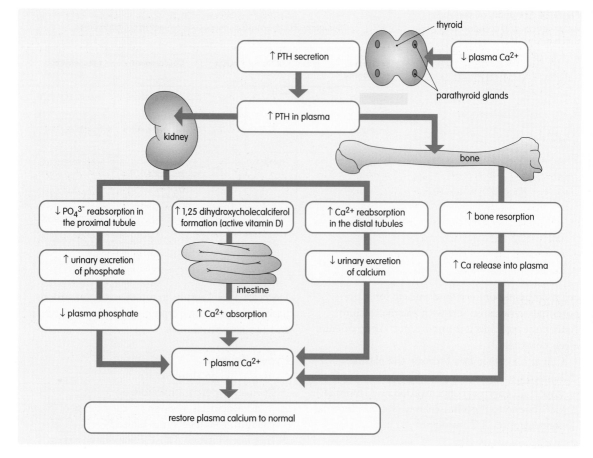

Fig. 3.25 Mechanisms of Ca^{2+} and phosphate homoeostasis. PTH, parathyroid hormone.

Ca^{2+} transport by the kidney

Only ionized Ca^{2+} is filtered through the glomerulus (approximately 50% plasma Ca^{2+}). Reabsorption proceeds as follows:

- Proximal tubule: 70% is reabsorbed by diffusion, Ca^{2+}-activated ATPase and the Ca^{2+}/Na^+ countertransport system.
- Thick ascending loop of Henle: 20–25% is reabsorbed passively.
- Distal convoluted tubule: 5–10% is reabsorbed against an electrochemical gradient.
- Collecting tubule: less than 0.5% is reabsorbed against an electrochemical gradient.

Calcium and phosphate homeostasis

Ca^{2+} and PO_4^{3-} concentrations are inversely proportional.

$$[Ca^{2+}] \times [PO_4^{3-}] = constant$$

Therefore, a rise in Ca^{2+} leads to a decrease in PO_4^{3-}, whereas a fall in Ca^{2+} stimulates an increase in PO_4^{3-} concentration, and vice versa.

Ca^{2+} and PO_4^{3-} enter the ECF via the intestine (diet) and bone stores. They leave the ECF via the kidneys (urine) and move into the bone.

Parathyroid hormone, vitamin D and calcitonin regulate Ca^{2+} and PO_4^{3-}.

Parathyroid hormone (PTH)

PTH is a polypeptide secreted by the parathyroid gland when there is a fall in plasma Ca^{2+}. PO_4^{3-} also affects PTH release, both directly and secondary to changes in Ca^{2+} levels. Figure 3.25 illustrates mechanisms of Ca^{2+} and PO_4^{3-} homeostasis. Vitamin D can also affect PTH release because it alters sensitivity of the parathyroid gland to Ca^{2+}.

Parathyroid hormone (PTH) secretion is stimulated by a decrease in [Ca^{2+}] and suppressed by a rise in [Ca^{2+}].

Vitamin D

Vitamin D refers to a group of closely related sterols obtained from the diet or by the action of ultraviolet light on certain provitamins. It is metabolized to 1,25-dihydroxycholecalciferol by the liver and kidney. This causes an increase in Ca^{2+} and PO_4^{3-} by:

- Enhancing intestinal absorption of Ca^{2+}.
- Increasing Ca^{2+} release from bone.
- Decreasing Ca^{2+} and PO_4^{3-} excretion.

Calcitonin

Calcitonin is a peptide produced by the parafollicular cells of the thyroid. It reduces Ca^{2+} release from bone causing a decrease in ECF Ca^{2+} concentration.

Phosphate

Phosphate is present in the plasma and interstitial fluid as:

- 'Acid' phosphate $H_2PO_4^{-}$.
- 'Alkaline' phosphate HPO_4^{3-}.

The proportion of the two forms depends on plasma pH. In cells, both inorganic forms (acid phosphate and alkaline phosphate) and organic forms (ATP, ADP and cAMP) are found. Plasma phosphate concentration is 0.8–1.3 mmol/L.

The kidney handles PO_4^{3-} as follows:

- Alkaline phosphate and acid phosphate are filtered by the glomerulus in a ratio of 4:1. Alkaline phosphate is converted to acid phosphate in the tubule as a result of H^+ secretion (see Fig. 3.20).
- 95% of the filtered PO_4^{3-} is reabsorbed in the early proximal tubule.
- Renal PO_4^{3-} excretion is increased by PTH, which is the only hormone to regulate phosphate transport.

Regulation of potassium and magnesium

Potassium (K⁺)

K^+ is the main intracellular cation. The intracellular and extracellular [K^+] is very important in the function of excitable tissues (e.g. nerves and muscles) as it determines the resting potentials of these tissues. Therefore, a constant [K^+] is critical for survival. Concentration is as follows:

- Total body K^+: 3–4 mmol/L.
- Intracellular fluid (ICF) K^+: 98%; 150–160 mmol/L.
- Extracellular fluid (ECF) K^+: 2%; 4–5 mmol/L.

- If extracellular [K^+] rises, the resting membrane potential is decreased (i.e. depolarized).
- If extracellular [K^+] falls, the resting membrane potential is increased (i.e. hyperpolarized).

Clinical features and causes of K⁺ disturbances

Hypokalaemia

Causes of a decreased K^+ concentration are:

- Vomiting.
- Diarrhoea.
- Diuretics.
- Excess insulin (e.g. Cushing's syndrome, steroids).
- Renal tubular acidosis.

Hypokalaemia is asymptomatic until K^+ concentration falls below 2–2.5 mmol/L. The low K^+ concentration results in a decreased resting potential (more negative) so the nerve and muscle cells become hyperpolarized. This means that cells are less sensitive to depolarizing stimuli and therefore less excitable, so fewer action potentials are generated and paralysis ensues. Clinical effects of hypokalaemia are:

- Muscle weakness, cramps and tetany, which starts in the lower extremities and progresses upwards (death is usually by paralysis of respiratory muscles).
- Impaired liver conversion of glucose to glycogen.
- Vasoconstriction and cardiac arrhythmias.
- Impaired ADH action, causing thirst and polyuria and no concentration of urine.
- Metabolic alkalosis due to an increase in intracellular H^+ concentration.

Treatment involves treating the underlying cause, and calculated oral or intravenous administration of potassium salt may be required.

Fig. 3.26 Potassium transport in the kidney.

Hyperkalaemia

Causes of an increased K^+ concentration are:

- Ingestion of K^+.
- Metabolic acidosis (diabetes mellitus).
- Insulin deficiency (i.e. Addison's disease).
- Excess cell breakdown (e.g. after cytotoxic cancer therapy).
- Renal failure.

Hyperkalaemia is asymptomatic until $K^+ > 6.5$ mmol/L. The increased K^+ concentration results in cell depolarization and increased excitability. The resting potential might be above the threshold potential, so cells cannot repolarize after an action potential, leading to paralysis. Death results from cardiac arrest due to the effects of hyperkalaemia on cardiac conduction. Fatal arrhythmias can occur when $K^+ > 7$ mmol/L.

Treatment involves:

- Dextrose and insulin to drive K^+ into cells.
- HCO_3^- to correct acidosis by stimulating K^+ entry into cells.
- Calcium salts to protect excitable tissues (of heart) against toxic effects of K^+.

- K^+ removal from body using loop diuretics, exchange resins (i.e. calcium resonium), and dialysis.

K^+ transport by the kidney

K^+ is filtered freely in the glomerulus. The proximal tubule reabsorbs 80–90%:

- Passively.
- Through tight junctions (paracellular movement).
- Via a concentration gradient.

In the distal tubule:

- K^+ reabsorption and leakage back are approximately equal in the early distal tubule.
- The late distal tubule and collecting ducts secrete K^+ into the urinary filtrate (passively via an electrochemical gradient) according to the body's needs—increased cellular K^+ concentration results in increased secretion and vice versa.

Changes in the distal tubular lumen also influence the rate of K^+ secretion. Figure 3.26 illustrates K^+ transport in the kidney.

ADH stimulates the secretion of K^+ by the collecting ducts by enhancing Na^+ reabsorption.

Aldosterone increases K^+ secretion. Increased plasma K^+ concentration stimulates aldosterone production by the adrenal cortex, so plasma aldosterone concentration rises. This in turn increases K^+ secretion and therefore K^+ excretion.

Magnesium (Mg^{2+})

Magnesium is an intracellular cation that:
- Controls mitochondrial oxidative metabolism and so regulates energy production.
- Is vital for protein synthesis.
- Regulates K^+ and Ca^{2+} channels in cell membranes.

The plasma concentration of magnesium is 2.12–2.65 mmol/L; about 20% is protein bound. Total body magnesium is 28 g, of which:
- 55% is in bone.
- 40% is in ICF.
- Up to 10% is in plasma at any one time.
- 0.6% is in ECF.

Clinical features and causes of Mg^{2+} disturbances
Hypomagnesaemia
Causes are:
- Decreased intake.
- Diarrhoea.
- Absorption disorder including fat absorption defects.
- Renal wasting—intrinsic (Bartter's syndrome), extrinsic (diuretics, e.g. thiazides).

Clinical features are non-specific. A fall in Mg^{2+} is followed by a decreased Ca^{2+}, but the mechanism for this is unknown.

Renal handling of Mg^{2+}
- In the glomerulus ionized Mg^{2+} (75% of total Mg^{2+}) is filtered.
- 15% is reabsorbed in the proximal tubule.
- 60% is reabsorbed in the thick ascending loop of Henle—the $Na^+/K^+/Cl^-$ cotransporter system enables Mg^{2+} absorption through the paracellular route. An Na^+/Mg^{2+} antiport and Mg^{2+} ATPase transport system also exists.
- Up to 5% is reabsorbed in the distal convoluted tubule.
- 0.5% is reabsorbed in the collecting tubule.

Regulation of Mg^{2+}

T_m for Mg^{2+} absorption is equal to the concentration of Mg^{2+} filtered. Therefore, an increase in Mg^{2+} results in increased filtering, which therefore exceeds the T_m, resulting in increased excretion.

There is intrinsic regulation by cells of the thick ascending loop of Henle—if Mg^{2+} decreases, cell transport of Mg^{2+} increases.

PTH increases reabsorption of Mg^{2+} in the thick ascending loop of Henle.

Regulation of erythropoiesis

Erythropoietin (EPO) is a glycoprotein hormone involved in erythrocyte production by the bone marrow. Although it is produced in the liver, the main sources of EPO (over 80%) are the kidney mesangial cells and renal tubular cells. The kidneys secrete EPO in response to hypoxia, which can develop in chronic states such as anaemia, in an attempt to increase the number of circulating red blood cells and therefore reduce hypoxia. This response is thought to be prostaglandin (PG) mediated, the PG stimulating the mesangial cells and renal tubular cells to synthesize EPO. EPO-sensitive stem cells are converted into proerythroblasts and then into red blood cells.

Patients with chronic renal failure often have a defective EPO production, leading to a normocytic normochromic anaemia. This can be treated by administration of exogenous (synthetic) EPO, which is produced using recombinant DNA technology. Subcutaneous or intravenous injections three times a week are required at a dose of 30–50 U/kg to reach a haemoglobin (Hb) count of 10–12 g/dL without the need for blood transfusions.

Iron deficiency is the most common cause of failure in EPO treatment, and is corrected with oral or intravenous supplements. Other reasons for failure include bleeding, malignancy and infection.

The complications of treatment are thrombotic complication, hypertension and fitting. These are associated with rapid increases in Hb concentration and haematocrit.

- Define clearance. Explain how it is measured and what its units are.
- Explain the relevance of clearance ratios.
- Describe how to measure the GFR and RBF. Discuss how this varies with age.
- Outline the factors that affect creatinine clearance.
- Define autoregulation and explain how it is achieved.
- Explain what osmoreceptors are, where they are located and what their function is.
- Briefly describe the synthesis, storage and function of ADH.
- Describe how the kidneys' ability to concentrate or dilute urine is altered in disease.
- Summarize the importance of the renin–angiotensin–aldosterone system.
- Outline the mechanisms controlling Na^+ reabsorption.
- Describe the effective circulating volume and explain how this is regulated.
- List the causes and the clinical presentation of SIADH.
- Distinguish the two types of diabetes insipidus and explain how they differ.
- State the normal pH range. Outline how and why it is tightly controlled.
- Explain what a 'buffer' is. Name the main buffering system in the body and describe how it works.
- Explain how metabolic acidosis and metabolic alkalosis are differentiated by arterial blood gas results and outline how you would correct each of them.
- Discuss the significance of the anion gap.
- Describe the distribution of K^+ within the body compartments and explain why it is important to keep this distribution constant.
- Explain the relationship between plasma calcium and phosphate. Describe the influence of three factors involved in their regulation.
- Discuss when erythropoietin release is stimulated and what its effects are.

4. The Kidneys in Disease

Congenital abnormalities of the kidney

Congenital structural abnormalities can develop within the kidney, as described below.

Agenesis of the kidney

Absence (agenesis) of the kidney can be unilateral or bilateral. Unilateral agenesis occurs in 1 in 1000 of the population. Agenesis occurs if the collecting system (from the ureteric buds) fails to fuse with the nephrons (from the metanephric mesoderm). The only kidney present gradually hypertrophies and is often abnormal with malrotation, ectopia or hydronephrosis. The kidney is at risk of infection and trauma. This disorder is associated with other developmental abnormalities such as absent testes or ovaries, spina bifida and congenital heart disease. Bilateral agenesis occurs in less than 1 in 3000 pregnancies and is incompatible with life. It is also known as Potter's syndrome, which is associated with pulmonary hypoplasia and oligohydramnios in utero. There is no treatment.

Potter's syndrome is characterized by renal agenesis, leading to oligohydramnios and hypoplastic lungs. The infant has low-set ears, a flattened nose and wide-set eyes.

Hypoplasia

The kidneys develop inadequately and are consequently smaller than average. This is a rare disorder, affecting one or both kidneys, which are prone to infection and stone formation.

Ectopic kidney

The incidence of ectopic kidney is 1 in 800. The kidney does not ascend fully into the abdomen, so remains lower than usual (if it remains in the pelvis, it is called a 'pelvic kidney'—Fig. 4.1). It is usually unilateral and, the lower the kidney, the more abnormal it is. As a result of the abnormal positioning, the ureters can be obstructed by neighbouring structures, leading to obstructive uropathy, infection and stone formation. This disorder can also affect pregnancy and birth.

Horseshoe kidney

The incidence of horseshoe kidney is between 1 in 600 and 1 in 1800, and is more common in boys than girls. The two kidneys fuse across the midline, usually at their lower poles, by renal tissue or a fibrous band (Fig. 4.2). The horseshoe kidney is usually lower than normal because the inferior mesenteric artery limits its ascent. It can also be malrotated and is prone to reflux, obstruction, infection and stone formation.

Cystic diseases of the kidney

Overview

Cystic diseases of the kidney form a spectrum of diseases comprising hereditary, developmental (but not hereditary) and acquired disorders. They can result if the ureteric bud or kidney tissue fails to develop. Some of these diseases can lead to chronic renal failure (CRF). Diagnosis is made by finding multiple cysts on ultrasound. A single simple cyst is not an uncommon finding and should be considered normal.

Cystic renal dysplasia

This is an area of undifferentiated mesenchyme or cartilage within the parenchyma. It can be unilateral (better prognosis) or bilateral, and is often associated with obstructive abnormalities in the ureter and lower urinary tract. Presentation is in childhood as an abdominal mass, treated with surgical excision.

Polycystic kidney disease
Adult—autosomal dominant
Incidence and presenting features
This type of polycystic kidney disease accounts for 8–10% of chronic renal failure. Inheritance is

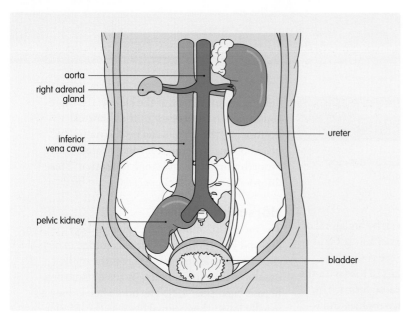

Fig. 4.1 Ectopic (pelvic) kidney.

aorta

right adrenal
gland

inferior
vena cava

pelvic kidney

ureter

bladder

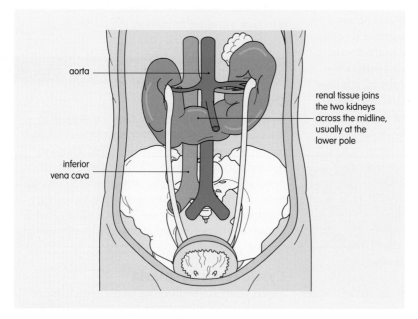

aorta

inferior
vena cava

renal tissue joins
the two kidneys
across the midline,
usually at the
lower pole

Fig. 4.2 Horseshoe kidney.

autosomal dominant and three polycystic kidney disease (PKD) genes have been identified:

- PKD 1: on chromosome 16 (accounts for 85% of cases).
- PKD 2: on chromosome 4 (accounts for 10% of cases).
- PKD 3: accounts for a minority of cases and has yet to be mapped.

These mutations are thought to alter tubular epithelium growth and differentiation. Presentation is at 30–40 years of age with hypertension, urinary symptoms or bilateral large palpable kidneys. End-stage renal failure can develop, usually in the 5th or 6th decade of life.

Pathology
Cysts develop anywhere in the kidney, when dilatations in the nephron (Fig. 4.3A) compress the surrounding parenchyma and impair renal function. Sites for cyst formation are:

Fig. 4.3 Polycystic adult (A) and childhood (B) kidney disease.

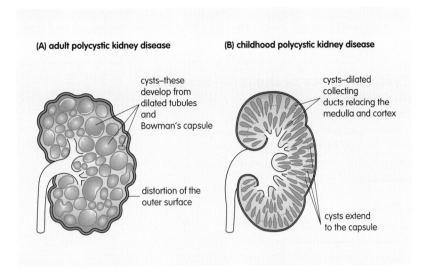

(A) adult polycystic kidney disease

cysts–these develop from dilated tubules and Bowman's capsule

distortion of the outer surface

(B) childhood polycystic kidney disease

cysts–dilated collecting ducts relacing the medulla and cortex

cysts extend to the capsule

- Both kidneys.
- Liver (lined by biliary epithelium) in 30–40% of cases.
- Pancreas, lungs, ovaries, spleen and other organs.

Complications include uraemia, hypertension and berry aneurysms (found in 10–20% of cases). These develop as a result of congenital weakness in the arteries and increased blood pressure; they can lead to a subarachnoid or cerebral haemorrhage.

Macroscopically, the kidneys are large with clear yellow fluid-filled cysts replacing the parenchyma. Haemorrhage into the cysts can occur. Microscopically, the cysts are lined by cuboidal epithelium.

Diagnosis
Diagnosis is made by:
- Ultrasound or computerized tomography (CT): this shows bilateral enlarged kidneys with multiple cysts.
- Genetic testing in families known to carry the PKD gene.

Prognosis
Morbidity and mortality are often the result of hypertension, for example myocardial infarction and cerebrovascular disease. The condition also leads to CRF. Rarely, complications are produced by the extrarenal cysts.

Treatment
This involves controlling blood pressure. Dialysis and renal transplant are needed if CRF develops.

Child—autosomal recessive
Incidence and presenting features
This rare condition presents with enlarged kidneys, or stillbirth. Both sexes are affected equally and more than one gene might be involved.

Pathology
Macroscopically, large kidneys with a radial pattern of fusiform-like cysts ('sunburst pattern') are seen. Both kidneys are enlarged by multiple dilated collecting ducts which form the cysts. These replace the medulla and cortex and extend into the capsule (see Fig. 4.3B). The liver is almost always affected, with cysts, bile duct cell proliferation, fibrosis interfering with liver function and eventual portal hypertension.

Diagnosis, prognosis and treatment
Diagnosis is based on the presence of a palpable mass and ultrasound findings. Treatment involves managing the renal failure, hypertension and respiratory problems.

The prognosis is poor and death usually occurs due to renal or respiratory failure within the first few weeks of life, unless renal replacement therapy is given. Some children can survive for several years with independent renal function and develop portal hypertension and hepatic fibrosis.

Cystic diseases of the renal medulla
Medullary sponge kidney
Incidence and presenting features
This is uncommon (1 in 20000). It usually presents at 30–40 years of age with symptoms of urinary tract infection (UTI), stone formation or haematuria.

Pathology
Dilated collecting ducts in the medulla result in multiple cyst formation, mainly in the papillae (Fig. 4.4). Small calculi can develop within the cysts. One, part of one, or both kidneys can be affected. Macroscopically, some cysts are seen extending into the medulla from the involved calyces. In severe cases, the medulla looks spongy.

Diagnosis, prognosis and treatment
Diagnosis is by intravenous urography (IVU). The prognosis is good, with renal function remaining intact. A partial nephrectomy might be required.

Nephronophthisis
Incidence and presenting features
This is an autosomal recessive condition that presents by the age of 25. Clinical features are polydipsia, polyuria, growth retardation and eventual renal failure. The disorder can coexist with retinal degeneration, optic atrophy, retinitis pigmentosa (giving tunnel vision), Laurence–Moon–Biedl syndrome or congenital hepatic fibrosis.

Pathology
Macroscopically, the kidneys appear small and fibrosed. Microscopically, there is interstitial inflammation and tubular atrophy. Later, multiple small medullary cysts develop.

Diagnosis, prognosis and treatment
Diagnosis is made from the family history and renal biopsy (this shows chronic tubulointerstitial nephritis). The disorder results in progressive renal failure, and treatment involves dialysis and renal transplant.

Acquired cystic disease (ACD) (dialysis-associated)
ACD occurs in patients with CRF who have received dialysis for some time. The damaged

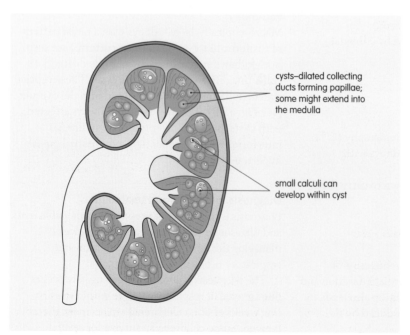

cysts–dilated collecting ducts forming papillae; some might extend into the medulla

small calculi can develop within cyst

Fig. 4.4 Medullary sponge kidney.

kidneys develop many small cysts throughout the cortex and medulla, caused by obstruction of the tubules by interstitial fibrosis. The cysts have an atypical hyperplastic epithelial lining that can undergo malignant change.

Simple cysts

These are very common, with incidence increasing with age. They vary in size (usually 2–5cm in diameter) and number, and contain clear fluid. Microscopically, they have a cuboidal epithelial lining and a thin capsule. Renal function is not affected but pain might be felt if there is haemorrhage into the cyst. The cysts can be differentiated from tumours by ultrasound (solid mass versus cystic mass).

Diseases of the glomerulus

Overview

Glomerular disease (usually called glomerulonephritis—GN) can be classified as:
- Hereditary (e.g. Alport's and Fabry's syndromes).
- Primary (most common): disease process originates from the glomerulus.
- Secondary to systemic diseases: e.g. diabetes mellitus, systemic lupus erythematosus (SLE), bacterial endocarditis.

Four structures within the glomerulus are prone to damage:
- Capillary endothelial cell lining.
- Glomerular basement membrane.
- Mesangium supporting the capillaries.
- Podocytes on the outer surface of the capillary.

Hereditary glomerular disease
Alport's syndrome

This is usually X-linked, affecting mainly males (females are usually asymptomatic carriers). Autosomal dominant and autosomal recessive patterns of inheritance have also been described. An abnormality of basement membrane collagen IV is found in all patients, and they lack the Goodpasture's antigen.

Presentation is with glomerulonephritis with haematuria, ocular abnormalities and sensorineural deafness. Ocular lesions include lens dislocation, cataract and conical cornea. It is also associated with platelet dysfunction and hyperproteinaemia.

A few patients develop end-stage renal failure in childhood and adolescence. Females might have microscopic haematuria, but rarely develop end-stage renal failure. Treatment involves dialysis and/or transplantation.

Fabry's syndrome

This is a rare X-linked disorder, with a glycolipid metabolism defect due to the deficiency of galactosidase A. As a result, ceramide trihexoside (a glycosphingolipid) accumulates and is deposited in the kidneys, skin and vascular system. This disorder is associated with cardiac problems such as angina and cardiac failure—consequently, most patients die in the 5th decade of life.

Clinical manifestations of glomerular disease

Glomerular disease usually presents in one of the following five ways (Fig. 4.5):
- Asymptomatic haematuria and proteinuria.
- Acute nephritic syndrome.
- Rapidly progressive glomerular disease.
- Nephrotic syndrome.
- Chronic renal failure (CRF).

Glomerular disease is classified as:
- Focal—affects only some glomeruli.
- Diffuse—affects all the glomeruli.
- Segmental—affects only part of the glomerulus.
- Global—affects the entire glomerulus.

Asymptomatic haematuria

Haematuria due to glomerular disease is often painless and can be continuous or intermittent. Primary and secondary causes are summarized in

Summary of types of glomerular disease and their clinical presentations		
Clinical presentation	Primary glomerular cause	Secondary cause
asymptomatic haematuria	mesangial IgA glomerulonephritis (GN); other GN; exercise-induced haemoglobinuria	Henoch–Schönlein purpura (HSP); systemic lupus erythematosus (SLE); bacterial endocarditis
asymptomatic proteinuria	mesangial capillary GN; any other GN; focal segmental glomerulosclerosis; shunt nephritis; any cause of renal scarring	HSP; SLE; bacterial endocarditis; polyarteritis nodosa (PAN); severe long-standing hypertension; pregnancy
acute nephritic syndrome	post-streptococcal GN; non-streptococcal GN; rapidly progressive GN; focal proliferative GN; mesangial IgA GN	SLE; microscopic polyangiitis (microscopic PAN); Wegener's granulomatosis
nephrotic syndrome	minimal change disease; membranous glomerulonephropathy; membranoproliferative GN; focal segmental glomerulosclerosis; shunt nephritis (rare)	HSP; SLE; tumour; amyloid; diabetes mellitus; drugs (e.g. penicillamine, gold); bacterial endocarditis; congenital nephrotic syndrome
chronic renal failure glomerulosclerosis	this develops as a long-term consequence of any of the above diseases	

Fig. 4.5 Summary of types of glomerular diseases and their clinical presentations.

Fig. 4.5. It should be noted that heavy exercise can result in haemoglobinuria (not haematuria).

Asymptomatic proteinuria
This is characterized by proteinuria (usually 0.3–3g protein daily) with no other symptoms. Possible causes are summarized in Fig. 4.5.

Acute nephritic syndrome
The symptoms and signs of acute nephritic syndrome are:
- Oliguria/anuria.
- Hypertension.
- Fluid retention—seen as facial oedema.
- Haematuria—microscopic or macroscopic.
- Uraemia.
- Proteinuria.

Patients might also complain of loin pain, headache and general malaise. Primary and secondary causes of acute nephritic syndrome are summarized in Fig. 4.5.

Rapidly progressive GN (RPGN)
RPGN, or crescentic GN, occurs when there is severe glomerular injury. It presents with haematuria, oliguria and hypertension, eventually causing renal failure.

Nephrotic syndrome
This is characterized by proteinuria (typically >3g/24h), hypoalbuminaemia and oedema. Hyperlipidaemia is also present. Primary and secondary causes are summarized in Fig. 4.5.

Chronic renal failure (CRF)

CRF results from any disease causing progressive nephron loss. The kidney shrinks, with cortical thinning. Most of the glomeruli consist of hyaline balls, with almost complete tubular atrophy. This is often asymptomatic in the early stages. Later, symptoms develop as waste products accumulate and erythropoietin or vitamin D production is reduced. Symptoms include:

- Uraemia.
- Hypertension.
- Salt and water retention causing oedema.
- Anaemia.
- Nausea, vomiting, diarrhoea.
- Gastrointestinal bleeding.
- Itching.
- Polyuria and nocturia.
- Lethargy.
- Paraesthesiae (due to polyneuropathy).
- Mental slowing and clouding of consciousness (terminal stage).

In extreme cases, oliguria results. The only treatment is dialysis until renal transplantation is possible.

The mechanisms of glomerular injury
In situ immune-complex deposition

Antigen–antibody immune complexes form within the kidney when antibodies react with intrinsic or planted antigens within the glomerulus (Fig. 4.6A).

Antiglomerular basement membrane (anti-GBM) disease is an example of reaction to intrinsic antigens. Antibodies are formed against an antigen in the GBM, to form a complex which stimulates the complement cascade. This damages the glomerulus and leads to rapidly progressing renal failure. The anti-GBM antibodies also attack the basement membrane of the alveoli in the lungs. The triad of anti-GBM antibodies, GN and pulmonary haemorrhage is known as Goodpasture's syndrome.

Reaction to planted antigens occurs when circulating antigens are deposited within the glomerulus. They can be:

- Exogenous: e.g. bacteria such as group A β-haemolytic streptococci, which cause post-streptococcal GN. Other antigens include bacterial products (endostreptosin), aggregated IgG, viruses, parasites and drugs.
- Endogenous: e.g. anti-DNA antibodies react with circulating DNA (as seen in SLE).

Circulating immune complex nephritis

This is the most common mechanism of immune-mediated damage. Immune complexes form outside the kidney and become trapped in the glomerulus after travelling to the kidney via the renal circulation (Fig. 4.6B). The antigen can be:

- Exogenous: bacteria (e.g. group A streptococci such as *Treponema pallidum*), surface antigen of hepatitis B, hepatitis C virus antigen, tumour antigens, viruses.
- Endogenous: DNA in SLE.

When trapped in the glomerulus, the immune complexes activate the classic complement pathway, causing acute inflammation of the glomerulus. Immunofluorescence microscopy shows neutrophil deposits along the basement membrane and/or in the mesangium. These increase vascular permeability.

Cytotoxic antibodies

Antibodies to glomerular cell antigens cause damage without the formation and deposition of immune complexes (Fig. 4.6C). This is uncommon. An example would be antibody fixing to mesangial cells, resulting in complement-mediated mesangiolysis and mesangial cell proliferation.

Cell-mediated immunity

Sensitized T cells from cell-mediated immune reactions play a role in the progression of acute GN to chronic GN (Fig. 4.6D). Glomerular damage is thought to be mediated by macrophages and T lymphocytes.

Activation of alternative complement pathway

Bacterial polysaccharides, endotoxins, and IgA aggregates can stimulate the alternative complement pathway—the products of which deposit in the glomeruli, impairing glomerular function (Fig. 4.6E). This occurs in membranoproliferative GN.

A in situ immune complex deposition

glomerulus

Ab

Ag

IC

Bowman's capsule

B circulating immune complex nephritis

IC

IC

C cytotoxic antibodies

Ab

Ag

damage without deposits

D cell-mediated immunity

sensitized T cell

damage

E activation of alternative complement pathway

bacterial polysaccharides, endotoxin, IgA aggregates

Factor B → C3 ← magnesium

← Factor D

C3bBb (C3 convertase)

broken down
Factor I
and
Factor H

stabilized
by properdin
C3NeF
(C3 nephritic
factor in the body)

C3 → C3b

C3b and other components

damage

Fig. 4.6 The five mechanisms of immune complex renal disease. Ab, antibody; Ag, antigen; IC, immune complex.

Acute glomerulonephritis (GN)
Post-streptococcal GN
This presents 1–3 weeks following a group A β-haemolytic streptococcal infection of the tonsils, pharynx or skin. Clinical features include proteinuria, haematuria and a low GFR (this causes fluid retention, oligaemia and hypertension). All the glomeruli are involved thus resulting in a diffuse proliferative GN—'proliferative' because there is an increase in the cellularity in the glomerulus. Treatment is usually conservative, with antibiotics to treat any remaining infection. The prognosis is excellent in children but only 60% of adults recover completely; the rest develop hypertension or renal impairment.

Non-streptococcal GN
Non-streptococcal GN follows a similar process to that for post-streptococcal GN except that the causative organism is not streptococcus. It can be triggered by:
- Other bacteria (i.e. staphylococci and pneumococci).
- Parasites (*Toxoplasma gondii*, Plasmodium).
- Viruses.

Both acute and chronic GN increase BP and decrease GFR. However, patients with acute GN also have oedema.

Rapidly progressive (crescentic) glomerulunephritis (RPGN)
This is seen when there is severe glomerular injury. Histologically, glomerular injury results in leakage of fibrin, which stimulates epithelial cells and macrophages within the Bowman's capsule to proliferate and form crescent-shaped masses, reducing glomerular blood supply. It can be seen as part of systemic illnesses such as SLE, Wegener's granulomatosis and microscopic polyangiitis. As the name suggests, the disease progresses very rapidly and there is a loss of renal function within days to weeks. Thus, prompt diagnosis and treatment is required to prevent hypertension, kidney scarring and renal failure Treatment is high-dose steroids, immunosuppressants and plasma exchange.

Nephrotic syndrome
This results when the glomerulus capillary wall is excessively permeable to plasma protein. This leads to heavy proteinuria (>3g/24h). The capillary wall becomes permeable to proteins of higher molecular weight as the severity of injury increases. Heavy proteinuria leads to low plasma albumin and therefore tissue oedema. The management and complications of nephrotic syndrome are discussed later in this chapter (p. 89).

Minimal change disease
This is the most common cause of nephrotic syndrome in children under the age of six, and more commonly affects males. No significant renal changes are seen under the light microscope (hence the name). Under the electron microscope there is podocyte fusion, i.e. foot process effacement. The cause is unknown, but potential mechanisms include a postallergic reaction, circulating immune complexes, or altered T-cell immunity. Treatment involves corticosteroid therapy and cyclosporin or cyclophosphamide (if resistant). The prognosis is good in children and variable in adults, but usually good. Occasionally, this disorder causes end-stage renal failure.

Membranous glomerulonephropathy
This is a chronic disease characterized by:
- Subepithelial deposition of immune complexes.
- Basement membrane thickening.

It accounts for 40% of adult nephrotic syndrome and is more common in males. Causes are idiopathic (85%), primary or secondary. Secondary causes include:
- Infections: syphilis, malaria, hepatitis B.
- Tumours: melanoma, carcinoma of the bronchus, lymphoma.
- Drugs: penicillamine, heroin, mercury, gold.
- Systemic illnesses: SLE.

Histology reveals widespread glomerular basement thickening caused by immunoglobulin deposition.

Over time, the abnormal excess mesangial matrix causes hyalinization of the glomerulus and death of individual nephrons. Drug treatment involves corticosteroids, cyclophosphamide, ciclosporin and chlorambucil. Prognosis depends on the cause; 30% of idiopathic cases develop CRF and require dialysis or transplantation. In secondary membranous glomerulonephropathy, treatment of underlying disease causes disease remission. Complications of membranous glomerulopathy are the same as those for nephrotic syndrome (see page 89).

- Membranous GN is the most common cause of nephrotic syndrome in older patients.
- Minimal change GN is the most common cause of nephrotic syndrome in children.

Membranoproliferative glomerulonephropathy

This is common in children and young adults, and more common in females than males. It is characterized histologically by diffuse global basement membrane thickening and mesangial proliferation. It is usually primary, but can be secondary to disorders such as SLE and malaria. Primary membranoproliferative GN is classified as:

- Type I (more common): immune complexes deposit in the subendothelium, causing inflammation and capillary thickening. This occurs in infections, tumours, drug reactions, genetic disorders, connective tissue disorders (e.g. SLE) and complement deficiencies.
- Type II: caused by activation of the alternative complement pathway (dense deposit disease [DDD]) following an infection. Histology reveals thickened capillaries caused by C3 deposition. It is associated with partial lipodystrophy.

Clinically, types I and II are indistinguishable, presenting with asymptomatic haematuria or combined nephrotic/nephritic syndrome. Prognosis is poor—the disease progresses to end-stage renal failure. Treatment involves dialysis and renal

transplantation. Recurrence occurs following transplant, particularly in type II disease.

Focal segmental glomerulosclerosis (FSGS)

This accounts for 10% of childhood and 15% of cases of adult nephrotic syndrome. It is more common in males and its causes are:

- Altered cellular immunity.
- Intravenous heroin use.
- AIDS.
- Reaction to chronic proteinuria.
- Idiopathic.

Histology reveals focal collapse and sclerosis, with hyaline deposits in glomerular segments. Presentation is with proteinuria or nephrotic syndrome, later developing haematuria and hypertension. Most develop CRF within 10 years. Treatment of the idiopathic form involves steroids, cyclophosphamide, cyclosporin, dialysis and renal transplantation. Recurrence can be seen after a renal transplant.

Focal proliferative GN

Focal proliferative GN results in inflammation of some parts of some glomeruli. Its presentation is less acute. It might affect only the kidney (IgA nephropathy, see below) or be secondary to systemic illnesses such as Henoch–Schönlein purpura (HSP), Goodpasture's syndrome, subacute bacterial endocarditis, vasculitis and other connective tissue diseases (e.g. SLE). Treatment with immunosuppression can be effective. The prognosis is variable. Necrotizing GN is also often seen in malignant hypertension.

IgA nephropathy (Berger's disease)

This is the most common primary glomerular disease worldwide, causing recurrent haematuria. There is some association with geographical location (more common in France, Australia and Singapore) and human leucocyte antigen (HLA) DR4. It typically affects young men after an upper respiratory tract infection. Presentation is with microscopic haematuria and proteinuria and renal impairment. There is hypertension and plasma IgA levels are raised. Histologically, IgA and C3 deposits are seen in the mesangium of all the glomeruli, with some mesangial proliferation (this is similar to histology seen in HSP). Eventually, there is sclerosis of the damaged segment. There is no effective treatment. Patients with late onset, proteinuria, increased blood pressure and increased creatinine at presentation have a worse prognosis—up to 20% of patients develop end-stage renal failure.

Chronic GN

This is diffuse global glomerular destruction and hyalinization associated with CRF. The kidneys are small with granular scarring. Chronic GN is the end-stage result of several types of GN, in particular, RPGN, focal glomerulosclerosis, membranoproliferative GN and IgA nephropathy. Histology reveals:

- Glomeruli hyalinization.
- Tubular atrophy.
- Interstitial fibrosis.

Unlike chronic pyelonephritis, the pelvicalyceal system is unaffected in chronic GN.

Glomerular lesions in systemic disease

Systemic disorders can cause glomerular disease. They are usually:

- Immune complex mediated (e.g. SLE, HSP, bacterial endocarditis).
- Vascular (e.g. microscopic polyangiitis, Wegener's granulomatosis).
- Metabolic (e.g. diabetes mellitus, amyloidosis).
- Drug treatment (e.g. penicillamine, gold, captopril, phenytoin).
- Infections (e.g. hepatitis B, leprosy, syphilis, malaria).

Systemic lupus erythematosus (SLE)

SLE is an autoimmune vasculitis characterized by antinuclear antibodies and widespread immune-complex-mediated inflammation. It is more common

in females, Asians and if an individual is HLA B8, DR2 or DR3 positive. It is a relapsing and remitting condition, usually diagnosed between 30 and 40 years of age. It affects many systems and organs in the body, for example, the joints, skin, heart, lungs and the kidneys (75% of cases). The renal lesions are the most important clinically and affect prognosis. Glomerular changes vary from minimal involvement to diffuse proliferative disease with:

- Immune complex deposition in mesangium.
- Basement membrane thickening.
- Endothelial proliferation.

This results in focal or diffuse proliferative GN, or membranous glomerulopathy. Histologically, SLE is diagnosed by subendothelial deposition of immune complexes, which produce a characteristic wire-loop appearance. Patients present with proteinuria, oedema and hypertension. There may be extrarenal systemic symptoms. Patients may develop CRF, but the prognosis has been improved with immunosuppressive treatment (steroids, azathioprine or cyclophosphamide).

Henoch–Schönlein purpura (HSP)

HSP is seen predominantly in children, affecting males more than females. It is an immune-mediated systemic vasculitis that affects many parts of the body including:

- Skin: a purpuric rash is seen over on the extensor surface of the legs and arms and buttocks.
- Joints: resulting in pain.
- Intestine: resulting in abdominal pain, vomiting, bleeding.
- Kidney: resulting in GN (one-third of patients develop IgA nephropathy).

HSP can follow an upper respiratory tract infection. It has an excellent prognosis in children.

Bacterial endocarditis

Glomerular disease in bacterial endocarditis is caused by:

- Immune complex deposits in the glomerulus.
- Embolism-mediated infarction—emboli break away from the heart valves.

The main histological diagnoses are focal, segmental and diffuse proliferative GN. Presentation is with microscopic haematuria, fluid retention and renal impairment. Renal lesions resolve upon antibiotic therapy.

Diabetic glomerulosclerosis

Diabetes mellitus affects several organs including the kidneys, which are the most commonly and severely damaged organs in diabetes. It is the most common reason for CRF dialysis treatment in developed countries. Renal manifestations include nodular glomerulosclerosis (described later) and arteriosclerosis, including benign nephrosclerosis with hypertension (Fig. 4.7 presents a summary of the natural history of diabetes). Histological features can include:

- Thickening of the capillary basement membrane.
- Increase in the matrix of the mesangium.
- A diffuse or nodular pattern of glomerulosclerosis (also known as Kimmelstiel–Wilson syndrome).
- Arterial hyalinosis of both the afferent and efferent arterioles—this predisposes to vessel occlusion.

The arteries can also be affected (especially in type II diabetes) and severe atheroma in the renal artery leads to renal ischaemia and hypertension. Papillary necrosis is a recognized complication, especially in the presence of infection. Diabetic nephropathy presents with microalbuminuria, which increases progressively to nephrotic range proteinuria (i.e. >3g/24h). Consequently, GFR gradually declines, leading to CRF, which can be seen in 30% of cases of insulin-dependent type I diabetes mellitus. It is also associated with diabetic complications elsewhere (e.g. retinopathy in the eyes). Chronic renal damage as a result of diabetes is associated and accelerated by hypertension.

Treatment includes ACE inhibitors to reduce proteinuria (these are discussed later), strict blood pressure and glycaemic control and dialysis for end-stage renal failure.

Amyloidosis

This disorder involves deposition of amyloid (an extracellular fibrillar protein) in the glomeruli, usually within the mesangium and subendothelium, and sometimes in the subepithelial space. Deposits can also be found in the walls of the blood vessels and in the interstitium. Clinically, this results in heavy proteinuria or the nephrotic syndrome, eventually leading to CRF (due to ischaemia and glomerulosclerosis). Dialysis or transplant is required to prevent death from uraemia.

Goodpasture's syndrome

In Goodpasture's syndrome, autoantibodies to type IV collagen in the glomerular basement membrane

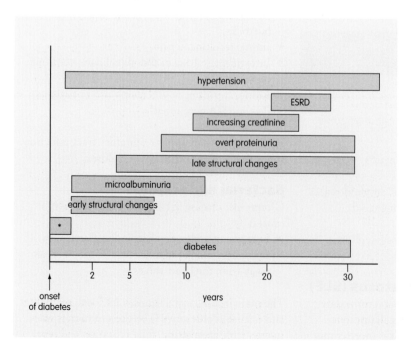

Fig. 4.7 Summary of the natural history of diabetes. *indicates functional changes in kidney size (increased) and short-term glomerular filtration rate (increased). ESRD, end-stage renal disease.

develop, causing inflammation. Presentation is with a rapidly progressive 'crescentic' GN with acute renal failure and lung haemorrhage. Prognosis is poor without treatment, which involves:
- Plasma exchange (to remove the antibodies).
- Corticosteroids (to reduce inflammation).

Microscopic polyarteritis nodosa (PAN; also known as microscopic polyangiitis)

This is a necrotizing vasculitis affecting the small arteries of the body; it is more common in males. Initially, there is a focal, segmental or necrotizing GN followed by RPGN. Histology reveals extensive necrosis, fibrin deposition and epithelial crescents. Microscopic PAN is associated with circulating antineutrophil cytoplasmic antibodies (ANCA), which complex with perinuclear antigen in fixed neutrophils (pANCA).

Wegener's granulomatosis

This is a rare necrotizing vasculitis affecting the nose, upper respiratory tract and kidneys. It typically presents between 40 and 50 years of age. The glomerular disease is similar to that for microscopic PAN, with granuloma formation. Presentation is with asymptomatic haematuria or nephritic syndrome (focal segmental GN) or RPGN. It is associated with ANCA, which characteristically recognizes a cytoplasmic antigen in fixed neutrophils (cANCA).

Hereditary nephritis

This is a spectrum of conditions, usually inherited, which present as GN with haematuria, often progressing to renal failure (e.g. Alport's syndrome, see p. 67).

Diseases of the tubules and interstitium

Overview

The tubules and interstitium are affected by several diseases. Typically, tubules become obstructed (this reduces glomerular filtration) or their transport functions become impaired (reduces water and solute reabsorption). Damage can be acute or chronic.

Acute tubular necrosis (ATN)

ATN is the result of acute tubular cell damage by ischaemia or toxins. It can be oliguric (<400mL/day urine) or non-oliguric. Hyperkalaemia can develop as a result of K^+ retention and this can trigger cardiac arrhythmias, which can be life-threatening. Uraemia develops because there is a significant fall in GFR—this could be due to haemodynamic changes and intratubular obstruction. Recovery is accompanied by a diuretic phase that occurs because of failure to concentrate urine (this can cause hypokalaemia).

ATN is a cause of acute renal failure (ARF). Mortality is up to 50% but full recovery is possible with prompt treatment—fluid and electrolyte therapy and dialysis if necessary.

Ischaemic ATN

This is caused by hypotension and hypovolaemic shock following trauma, infections, burns or haemorrhage. There is a rapid fall in blood pressure, which causes hypoperfusion of the peritubular capillaries with consequent tubular necrosis along the entire length of the nephron. The kidneys appear pale and swollen. Histology reveals:
- Infiltration of inflammatory cells and the tubular cells.
- Flattened and vacuolated tubular cells.
- Interstitial oedema.
- Cellular debris and protein casts in the distal tubule and the collecting ducts.
- Myoglobin in the casts in crush injuries.

NSAIDs can increase the risk of ATN following other renal insults by preventing the synthesis of prostaglandins (PGs). PGs are vasodilators, which protect the kidney from ischaemic injury by dilating blood vessels and increasing blood flow.

Toxic ATN

This disorder is caused by agents with specific nephrotoxic activity causing damage to the epithelial cells. Such substances include:
- Organic solvents: carbon tetrachloride (CCl_4) in dry-cleaning fluid.
- Heavy metals (gold, mercury, lead, and arsenic).
- Antibiotics (gentamicin).
- Pesticides.

These substances cause the cells to come away from the basement membrane and consequently collect in and obstruct the tubular lumen. The effect is limited because there is regeneration of the epithelial cells in 10–20 days, which permits clinical recovery and is confirmed by the presence of mitotic figures on biopsy. Damage by nephrotoxic substances is limited to the proximal tubules. The kidneys appear swollen and red.

Tubulointerstitial nephritis
Urinary tract infection (UTI)
Incidence and risk factors
UTIs are very common. They can involve the bladder (cystitis) or the kidneys (pyelonephritis) or both. It is more common in boys in infancy because of congenital abnormalities; this reverses at puberty, with more females being affected thereafter because of urethral trauma and pregnancy. Women are particularly at risk of lower UTIs because they have a short urethra, but further investigation is required if infections are recurrent. Any UTI in children and adult males should be investigated to exclude an underlying renal tract abnormality. UTI rarely progresses to renal damage in adults if the renal tract is normal. Treatment involves a high fluid intake, regular bladder emptying and prophylactic antibiotics. After the age of 40, UTI is again more common in men because of prostatic disease, causing bladder outflow obstruction. Risk factors for UTIs include:

- Long-term catheterization.
- Diabetes mellitus.
- Lower urinary tract obstruction (congenital abnormalities or calculi).
- Pregnancy.
- Tumours.
- Immunosuppression.
- Vesicoureteric reflux.

Presentation
UTIs present silently (asymptomatic bacteriuria) or with dysuria (pain on passing urine), frequency and urgency of micturition. Involvement of the kidneys causes loin pain and fever.

Diagnosis
A diagnosis of UTI requires over 10^5 organisms/mL from a midstream urine specimen on culture. In the majority of UTIs the infecting organism comes from the patient's own faecal flora (Fig. 4.8).

Pyelonephritis
This is a bacterial infection of the kidney and results in inflammation and damage to the renal

Incidence of community- and hospital-acquired UTIs caused by bacteria		
Organism	Community (%)	Hospital (%)
Escherichia coli	80–90	45–55
Proteus	5–10	10–12
Klebsiella	1–2	15–20
Enterobacter	–	2–5
Pseudomonas	–	10–15
Acinetobacter	–	<1
coagulase-negative *Staphylococcus*	1–2	1–2
Staphylococcus aureus	–	<1
Enterococcus	<1	10–12

Fig. 4.8 Incidence of community- and hospital-acquired urinary tract infections (UTIs) caused by bacteria.

calyces, parenchyma and pelvis. It can be acute or chronic.

Acute pyelonephritis
This occurs because of infection in the kidney and is spread via two routes:

1. Ascending infection: bacteria from the gut enter the kidney from the lower urinary tract if there is an incompetent vesicoureteric valve. This permits vesicoureteric reflux (VUR) and results in ascending transmission of infection.
2. Haematogenous spread: seen in patients with septicaemia or infective endocarditis. The pathogens include fungi, bacteria (staphylococci and *Escherichia coli*) and viruses. The kidney is often affected in septicaemic diseases because of its large blood supply.

The predisposing factors of acute pyelonephritis are:

- Urinary tract obstruction (congenital and acquired).
- VUR.
- Instrumentation of the urinary tract.
- Sexual intercourse.
- Diabetes mellitus.
- Immunosuppression (HIV, lymphoma and transplants).

Patients present with general malaise, fever, loin pain, tenderness and often rigors with or without symptoms of lower UTI. Infection spreads into the renal pelvis and papillae and causes abscess formation throughout the cortex and medulla.

With retrograde ureteric spread the kidney characteristically contains areas of wedge-shaped suppuration especially at the upper and lower poles. In septicaemia there is haematogenous seeding within the kidney and minute abscesses are distributed randomly in the cortex. On histology there is:

- Polymorphic infiltration of the tubules.
- Interstitial oedema.
- Focal inflammation.

Uncomplicated cases resolve with antibiotic treatment and high fluid intake. The important complications of acute pyelonephritis are:

- Renal papillary necrosis.
- Perinephric abscesses.
- Pyonephrosis (obstruction of the pelvicalyceal system).
- Chronic pyelonephritis.
- Fibrosis and scarring.

Chronic pyelonephritis

This condition is characterized by long-standing parenchymal scarring, which develops from tubulointerstitial inflammation. It is the end-result of various pathological processes. There are two main types:

1. Obstructive: chronic obstruction (stones, tumours or congenital abnormalities) prevents pelvicalyceal drainage and increases the risk of renal infection. Chronic pyelonephritis develops because of recurrent infection.

2. Reflux nephropathy: this is the most common cause of chronic pyelonephritis. It is associated with VUR, which is congenital. The organisms enter the ascending portion of the ureter with refluxed urine as the valvular orifice is held open on contraction of the bladder during micturition. Reflux results from the abnormal angle at which the ureter enters the bladder wall (Fig. 4.9).

The disease process usually begins in childhood and has a silent, insidious onset. Reflux of urine into the renal pelvis occurs during micturition and this increases the pressure in the major calyces. The high intrapelvic pressure forces urine into the collecting ducts with intraparenchymal reflux further distorting the internal structure. This is most predominant at the poles of the kidney and results in deep irregular scars on the cortical surface. The tubulointerstitial inflammation heals with the formation of corticomedullary scars that overlie the deformed and

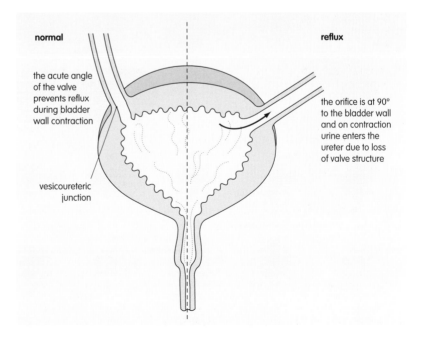

Fig. 4.9 Normal and refluxing (abnormal) junction.

dilated calyces, which are characteristic of chronic pyelonephritis (Fig. 4.10).

On histology there is interstitial fibrosis and dilated tubules containing eosinophilic casts; 10–20% of patients with CRF requiring dialysis have chronic pyelonephritis.

Diagnosis is made by intravenous pyelography (IVP) (see Chapter 8), which shows distortion of the calyceal system and contraction of the kidney because of cortical scarring. Generally, radiographs are avoided in children. Ultrasonography is also used to diagnose chronic pyelonephritis, but is less sensitive than IVP.

Toxin- and drug-induced tubulointerstitial nephritis

Heavy metals (mercury, gold, lead) and drugs (ampicillin, rifampicin, NSAIDs) can cause T-cell-mediated inflammation in the interstitium. This reaction usually occurs 2–40 days after exposure to the toxin. Clinical features include fever, skin rash, haematuria, proteinuria and acute renal failure (ARF). Withdrawal of the causative agent leads to recovery.

On histology there is interstitial oedema and tubular degeneration with eosinophil infiltration. In chronic analgesic abuse with phenacitin, and to a lesser extent aspirin, PG synthesis is inhibited, causing ischaemia (as described on p. 75 for

ischaemic ATN). This causes papillary necrosis and a secondary tubulonephritis (analgesic nephropathy). It is associated with an increased risk of developing transitional cell carcinomas with chronic analgesic abuse.

Papillary necrosis can be diagnosed by X-ray. It is seen in analgesic nephropathy, diabetes, sickle-cell disease and urinary tract obstruction.

Urate nephropathy

If there is an increased blood urate concentration, urate crystals are precipitated in the acidic environment of the collecting ducts, causing inflammatory obstruction and dilatation of the tubules. This eventually leads to fibrosis and atrophy. An increase in urate concentration can be caused by:

- Rapid cell turnover (e.g. in psoriasis or malignancy): in those patients with haematological or lymphatic malignancy who are receiving chemotherapy there is excess cell breakdown and release of nucleic acids, which results in acute urate nephropathy and ARF.

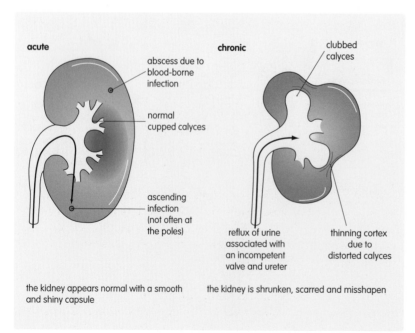

Fig. 4.10 Differences between acute and chronic pyelonephritis.

- Reduced uric acid clearance (e.g. in CRF): this is seen in patients with gout, in which there is a long-term deposition of urate in the kidney as a result of the constant high blood urate levels.

Urate nephropathy causes ARF or CRF depending on the time-course of urate deposition:
- Patients with malignancy treated with chemotherapy are prone to ARF.
- Patients with gout are prone to CRF.

Hypercalcaemia and nephrocalcinosis

A persistently high blood Ca^{2+} level causes Ca^{2+} deposition in the kidneys. The hypercalcaemia can be due to:
- Primary hyperparathyroidism.
- Multiple myeloma.
- Increased vitamin D activity.
- Bone metastases.

Renal insufficiency occurs in these patients because of stones (nephrolithiasis) or focal calcification in the renal parenchyma (nephrocalcinosis).

In nephrocalcinosis the Ca^{2+} accumulates in the tubular cells and the basement membrane, resulting in interstitial fibrosis and inflammation. Hypercalcaemia also causes a renal concentrating defect, which leads to polyuria, nocturia and dehydration.

Multiple myeloma

Approximately 50% of these patients develop renal insufficiency, which can cause ARF or CRF. Histological changes include:
- Bence-Jones proteins (light chains) enter the urine and these are toxic to the tubular epithelial cells. They combine with Tamm–Horsfall protein to precipitate as casts in the tubules, causing inflammation and obstruction to the tubular cells.
- Amyloid lambda (λ) or kappa (κ) light-chain fragments (paraproteins) are deposited in the renal blood vessels, glomeruli and tubules.
- Urate deposition (discussed above).
- Hypercalcaemia (discussed above).

Diseases of the renal blood vessels

Benign nephrosclerosis

This is the term given to the changes in renal vasculature in response to long-standing essential (benign) hypertension. The changes consist of hyaline arteriolosclerosis, which is characterized by thickening (due to hyperplasia of smooth muscle) and hyalinization (protein deposition) of the arteriolar wall. This causes narrowing of the lumen of the interlobular arteries, which functionally impairs the smaller branches. The changes are more severe in patients with systemic diseases that affect the renal vessels (e.g. diabetes). The vascular wall lesions gradually reduce the blood supply to the kidney, which leads to ischaemic atrophy of the nephrons. This accounts for the small, contracted and granular appearance of the kidneys seen in advanced cases of untreated essential hypertension. Renal function usually remains intact, although proteinuria is sometimes detected.

Malignant nephrosclerosis

This is associated with accelerated hypertension. It occurs in 1–5% of patients with hypertension. There is a sudden accelerated rise in blood pressure with an increase in diastolic pressure to over 130mmHg. In acute cases the kidney surface appears smooth and is covered in tiny petechial haemorrhages. There are fibrin deposits in the vessel wall, causing necrosis (fibrinoid necrosis), especially in the distal part of the interlobular arteries and the afferent arterioles.

Renal function is impaired because of the ischaemia that results from severe arterial damage. Patients have proteinuria and haematuria, which can occasionally be massive. Patients develop renal failure if untreated (in contrast to benign hypertension). Papilloedema is often present. The 5-year survival rate with treatment is 50%.

The trigger for the abrupt and rapid rise in blood pressure is unknown but might be associated with endothelial dysfunction. These patients also have increased plasma levels of renin, aldosterone and angiotensin.

Renal artery stenosis

Between 2 and 5% of hypertensive patients have hypertension secondary to renal artery stenosis

Contrasting clinical findings of fibromuscular dysplasia and atheromatous RAS		
	Fibromuscular dysplasia	Atheromatous RAS
age (years)	<40	>55
sex prevalence	F > M	M > F
bruit heard	80%	40%
vascular disease elsewhere	rare	common
renal failure	rare	well recognized
patient prognosis	good	poor

Fig. 4.11 Comparison between fibromuscular dysplasia and atheromatous renal artery stenosis (RAS).

(RAS) in one or both renal arteries. This is narrowing of the renal arteries caused by atheromatous plaques (70%) or fibromuscular dysplasia within the renal artery wall (Fig. 4.11). Poor renal perfusion is interpreted by the affected kidney as a fall in body fluid volume, which stimulates renin secretion. Ischaemia of the affected kidney leads to a small kidney.

Treatment options include:
- **Angioplasty:** to dilate the stenotic region. This can be supplemented with stenting to decrease the risk of restenosis.
- **Bypass surgery:** of the narrowed vessels. If the blood pressure is left uncontrolled the contralateral kidney may become damaged by hypertension.

Thrombotic microangiopathies

This is a group of diseases that are all characterized by necrosis and thickening of the renal vessel walls and thrombosis in the interlobular arterioles, afferent arterioles and glomeruli. All clinically present with a triad of:
- Haemolysis.
- Thrombocytopenia.
- Acute renal failure.

The main two microangiopathies are:
1. Haemolytic uraemic syndrome (HUS).
2. Thrombotic thrombocytopenic purpura (TTP).

Haemolytic uraemic syndrome (HUS)

This is characterized by the triad of:
- Microangiopathic haemolytic anaemia.
- Thrombocytopenia (decreased platelets).
- Renal failure (with normal clotting).

It is classified as:
- **Idiopathic:** this is more common in adults, and has a worse prognosis.
- **Secondary:** this can be associated with gastroenteritis (e.g. *Escherichia coli* 0157 toxin), drugs (oestrogen, ciclosporin A, cytotoxic therapy) or malignancy. HUS can also be caused by accelerated hypertension or, more rarely, there might be a genetic cause.

Clinical features include sudden onset of oliguria with haematuria—occasionally with malaena or haematemesis (usually if gastroenteritis is the cause)—and jaundice. Hypertension is seen in 50% of patients.

Treatment involves early supportive therapy with dialysis for renal failure. Fresh frozen plasma can be useful. Approximately 50% of patients later develop hypertension, and a few go on to develop chronic renal failure. Mortality ranges from 5 to 30%.

Thrombotic thrombocytopenic purpura (TTP)

This is a rare and idiopathic condition that is more common in females (usually <40 years) than in males. The features are fever, neurological signs (CNS involvement), haemolytic anaemia and thrombocytopenia. TTP has a similar disease process to HUS, but affects different sites. Renal involvement occurs in only 50% of cases, and presents with:
- Proteinuria.
- Haematuria.
- Renal insufficiency.

The majority of cases have a dominant CNS component, with thrombosis leading to ischaemia in the brain.

Histology shows thrombi consisting of fibrin and platelets in the terminal interlobular arteries, the afferent arterioles and glomerular capillaries.

Treatment involves corticosteroid therapy and plasma exchange.

Renal infarction
Embolic infarction
The embolus can come from:
- Thrombotic material from the left side of the heart.
- Atheromatous material from plaques.
- Bacterial vegetations from infective endocarditis.

The emboli lodge in the small renal vessels and cause narrowing of the arterioles and focal areas of ischaemic injury. It can be asymptomatic, or present with haematuria and loin tenderness. The areas of infarction appear pale and are characteristically wedge shaped.

Diffuse cortical necrosis
Diffuse cortical necrosis causes ARF and presents with anuria. This is a rare condition that results from profound hypertension caused by:
- Severe hypovolaemic shock.
- Sepsis.
- Eclampsia (pregnancy).

In response to hypotension, there is compensatory vasoconstriction that can cause infarction. This can be avoided by prompt resuscitation of the shocked patient. Once the disease is established, no agent has been shown to improve outcome. Prognosis is much better for focal infarction than for generalized cortical infarction. The surface of the kidney appears patchy with irregular yellow areas of necrosis, congestion and haemorrhage (limited to the outer part of the cortex). Infarcts can calcify over time.

Sickle-cell disease nephropathy
Thrombotic occlusion by deformed sickle-shaped red cells causes papillary necrosis. It is precipitated by cold, dehydration, infection and exercise. Presentation is with pain, haematuria and polyuria. Management involves analgesia, warmth and rehydration, blood transfusions and antibiotics (if infection is suspected).

Neoplastic disease of the kidney

Benign tumours of the kidney
These rarely cause symptoms and are usually found on autopsy.

Renal fibroma or hamartoma
This is the most common benign renal tumour. It is a small (less than 1cm diameter) firm, well-demarcated, white nodule in the medulla. The nodule is composed of spindle cells and collagen. It is often an incidental finding with clinical significance.

Cortical adenoma
This is a small (<3cm diameter) discrete, yellowish-grey tumour derived from renal tubular epithelium. It is an incidental finding in 20–25% of autopsies; it has a low malignant potential. On histology it is found to be composed of large vacuolated clear cells with small nuclei (this is also seen in renal cell carcinoma). Diagnosis depends on the size of the tumour:
- Less than 30mm diameter: benign adenoma.
- Over 30mm diameter: malignant carcinoma.

However, this grading is unreliable because small lesions could be growing carcinomas.

Angiomyolipoma ('hamartomatous malformation')
This is found in the cortex or medulla. The tumour is composed of blood vessels, smooth muscle and fat. Angiomyolipomas are associated with tuberous sclerosis, which is an inherited disease that involves the central nervous system, skin and other viscera.

Oncocytoma
This is an epithelial cell tumour that can grow to a diameter of 12cm but does not undergo malignant change. Histology reveals enlarged cells with a granular eosinophilic cytoplasm as a result of the vast number of mitochondria in the tumour cells.

Malignant tumours of the kidney
Renal cell carcinoma (RCC)
Incidence and risk factors
Approximately 90% of renal malignant tumours in adults are RCCs, which arise from the tubular epithelium. RCC is very rare in children and has a peak incidence in 60–70 year olds. The male to female ratio is 3:1. It has great geographical variance with the highest incidence in Scandinavia and the lowest in South America and Africa. Risk factors are:
- Acquired cystic disease in patients who require renal replacement therapy: RCC tends to occur at a much earlier age in these patients.
- Von Hippel–Lindau disease: this is a rare autosomal dominant condition caused by a

mutation on chromosome 25; 50–70% of these patients develop RCC.
- Smoking.

Presentation

Approximately 90% of cases present as haematuria. Non-specific symptoms include fatigue, weight loss and fever. There might be a mass in the loin. These are all late manifestations, presenting at an advanced stage of tumour progression, which is why prognosis is poor. RCC often metastasizes before local symptoms develop.

A small number of RCCs can secrete hormone-like substances such as:
- Parathyroid hormone (PTH), resulting in hypercalcaemia.
- Adrenocorticotrophic hormone (ACTH), resulting in a Cushing's-like syndrome.
- Erythropoietin, resulting in polycythaemia.
- Renin, resulting in hypertension.

As a result of these hormone-producing tumours, RCC commonly presents with paraneoplastic syndromes.

Diagnosis

Diagnosis is by:
- IVU: revealing a space-occupying lesion in the kidney that distorts the outline.
- Ultrasonography: distinguishes between solid and cystic lesions.
- Computed tomography (CT): provides preoperative staging (see Chapter 8).

Pathology

RCC consists of a yellow–brown, well-demarcated mass in the renal cortex, with a diameter of 3–15cm. Within this area there are patches of haemorrhage, necrosis and cyst formation. The tumours are most common at the upper pole of the kidney. The renal capsule is often intact, although it can be breached and the tumour will extend into the perinephric fat. Spread into the renal vein is often visible and rarely this extends into the inferior vena cava.

Histology reveals cells with clear cytoplasm that range from well differentiated to anaplastic.

Spread occurs by direct invasion of local tissues, via the lymph to lumbar nodes (one-third of cases), and via the blood (venous). Metastases are found in the lung, liver, bone, opposite kidney and adrenals.

Prognosis

Prognosis depends on tumour size and the degree of the spread; RCC staging involves assessing local, nodal and metastatic spread (TNM classification).
- T_1: confined to the kidney.
- T_2: enlarging tumour with distortion of the kidney with renal capsule intact.
- T_3: spread through the renal capsule into the perinephric fat with invasion into the renal vein.
- T_4: invasion into adjacent organs or the abdominal wall.
- N^+: lymph node involvement.
- M^+: metastatic spread.

Treatment

If there are no distant metastases, treatment involves a radical nephrectomy with removal of the associated adrenal gland, perinephric fat, upper ureter and the para-aortic lymph nodes. Postoperative radiotherapy is required to decrease risk of recurrence. There is little effective treatment available for metastatic disease. The average 5-year survival rate is 45%, increasing up to 70% if there is no metastatic disease at diagnosis.

Wilms' tumour (nephroblastoma)

Incidence and presentation

This is the most common malignant tumour in children. The peak incidence is in 1–4-year-olds, with both sexes affected equally. It is an embryonic tumour derived from the primitive metanephros. It presents with an abdominal mass and occasionally haematuria, abdominal pain and hypertension.

Pathology

The tumours are large solid masses of firm white tissue with areas of necrosis and haemorrhage. They often breach the renal capsule and grow into the perinephric fat. Histology reveals spindle cells or primitive blastema cells with epithelial and mesenchymal tissues, cartilage, bone and muscle. They are aggressive tumours, often presenting with metastatic disease of the lung.

Treatment and prognosis

Treatment involves nephrectomy, radiotherapy and chemotherapy. The long-term survival rate is over 80%.

Prognosis depends upon tumour size and distant spread at the time of diagnosis.

Urothelial carcinoma of the renal pelvis

This is a transitional cell tumour accounting for 5–10% of renal tumours. It can be caused by:

- Analgesic abuse.
- Exposure to aniline dyes used in the industrial manufacture of dyes, rubber and plastics.

Presentation with haematuria or obstruction occurs early, because the renal pelvis projects directly into the pelvicalyceal cavity.

Histology ranges from well-differentiated tumours to diffuse, invasive and anaplastic carcinomas. Poorly differentiated tumours have a poor prognosis and often invade the wall of the renal pelvis and the renal vein. Multiple tumours are also often found in the ureters and bladder. Fragments of papillary tumour and atypical tumour cells can be detected in the urine and this makes cytological diagnosis possible.

Metastases from lymphomas, lung or breast cancer or melanomas can deposit in the kidneys.

Figure 4.12 summarizes the common tumour sites throughout the urinary tract.

Renal responses to systemic disorders

Congestive cardiac failure (CCF)

CCF occurs when the pump mechanism of the heart cannot cope with its work load (i.e. providing the body with its metabolic requirements) so the cardiac output (CO) fails to perfuse the tissues adequately. This results in hypoperfusion of tissues and sodium and water retention. CCF is the common end result of all types of severe heart disease.

CCF can be caused by:
- Pump failure (low output heart failure).
- Increased demand (high output heart failure).

A normal heart can fail under high loads, but an abnormal heart will fail under normal loads.

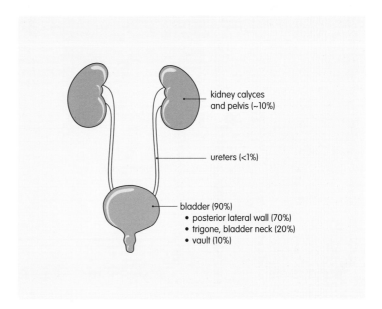

Fig. 4.12 Common tumour sites throughout the urinary tract.

A fall in CO leads to renal hypoperfusion. The kidney senses this as a sign of hypovolaemia and compensates by retaining NaCl and water to increase the circulating volume (Fig. 4.13). As the kidney attempts to increase the circulating fluid volume, peripheral oedema develops (left heart failure). This increases pulmonary venous pressure, stimulating fluid transudation from the capillaries in the lungs, which results in pulmonary oedema.

Treatment and management

Management involves reducing the fluid load within the body and thereby decreasing the workload of the heart.
• Diuretics: produce symptomatic relief from pulmonary oedema.
• Nitrates: produce venodilation, which decreases preload.
• Vasodilators (e.g. hydralazine): these reduce afterload.

• ACE inhibitors: act as vasodilators (by reducing the synthesis of angiotensin II) and as diuretics (by decreasing aldosterone synthesis).

Prognosis depends on the overall clinical picture, and the extent of cardiovascular disease. For further information refer to *Crash course: Cardiovascular system*.

Hypovolaemia and shock

Shock is a medical emergency in which the vital organs are hypoperfused as a result of either an inadequate circulating blood volume or heart failure. As the amount of oxygen and nutrients delivered to the cells is inadequate, the resulting hypoxic state within the cells leads to anaerobic metabolism and there is inefficient clearance of the metabolites, which build up in the cell. Hypovolaemia and mild shock cause tiredness, dizziness and a feeling of

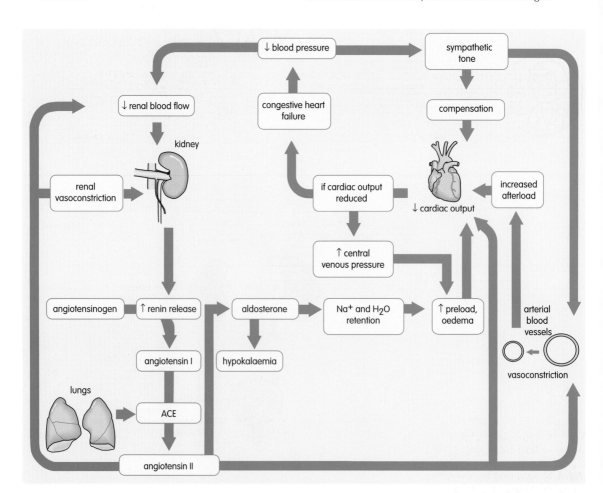

Fig. 4.13 Compensatory mechanisms in congestive cardiac failure (CCF). ACE, angiotensin-converting enzyme.

thirst. A severe decrease in the circulating volume stimulates sympathetic activity to maintain the blood pressure (BP) by:

- Tachycardia.
- Peripheral vasoconstriction.
- Increase in myocardial contractility.

Vasodilation occurs in the vital organs (heart, lungs, brain) to maintain blood supply, but this is at the expense of perfusion to other organs. If there is inadequate compensation, tissue hypoxia and necrosis can occur in vulnerable organs (e.g. acute tubular necrosis in the kidneys).

Types of shock
Cardiogenic shock
This occurs when the heart fails to maintain CO acutely (e.g. ischaemic heart disease, arrhythmias).

As a result, tissue perfusion decreases dramatically. Venous pressure increases, causing pulmonary or peripheral oedema (as described above). Prognosis is poor (90% mortality).

Hypovolaemic shock
This occurs when there is an acute reduction in effective circulating blood volume:

- Exogenous losses of plasma (e.g. burns), of blood (e.g. haemorrhage), or of water and electrolytes (e.g. diarrhoea and vomiting).
- Endogenous losses of fluid (e.g. sepsis and anaphylaxis).

Figure 4.14 shows the response to a fall in circulating fluid volume. To avoid excessive sympathetic activity in the kidneys (this results in vasoconstriction), more vasodilating prostaglandins (PGE_2 and PGI_2) are

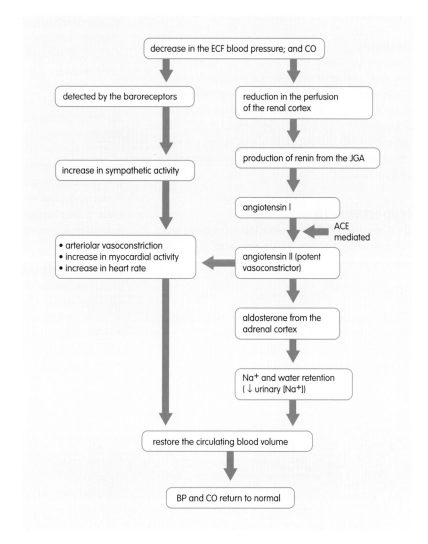

Fig. 4.14 Response to a fall in circulating fluid volume. ACE, angiotensin-converting enzyme; BP, blood pressure; CO, cardiac output; ECF, extracellular fluid; JGA, juxtaglomerular apparatus.

secreted within the kidneys. This maintains an adequate blood flow through the kidney to allow sufficient glomerular filtration, unless the shock is severe. The loss of large amounts of fluid has two major consequences:

- Volume depletion (decreases tissue perfusion).
- Electrolyte and acid–base disturbance.

As Na^+ is involved in the cotransport of H^+, K^+ and Cl^-, the acid–base balance is disturbed because Na^+ is retained. Cl^- is reabsorbed in equal quantities but, initially, there is increased secretion of H^+ and K^+, resulting in metabolic alkalosis (contraction alkalosis) and hypokalaemia. This is balanced by the shift to anaerobic metabolism as a result of hypoxia in the tissues, which eventually prevails to cause a metabolic acidosis. This is further potentiated as hypovolaemia becomes more severe, as less urine is excreted and H^+ is no longer excreted.

Treatment

Treatment of cardiogenic shock involves inotropes, whereas treatment of hypovolaemic shock requires fluid replacement to restore the extracellular volume. HCO_3^- is considered if there is severe acidosis (pH < 7.2) (see p. 54 for acid–base disturbances). If blood flow to the kidneys is not restored, renal failure results from tissue anoxia and necrosis.

Hypertension

BP is influenced by the interaction of genetic and environmental factors, which regulate CO and total peripheral resistance (TPR):

$$BP = CO \times TPR$$

The kidneys influence BP by regulating ECF volume. They also release vasoactive substances:

- Vasoconstrictors: angiotensin II.
- Vasodilators: prostaglandins.

Renal autoregulation maintains renal function despite variations in systolic BP. Any change in the ECF will affect the BP. The kidney compensates for these changes by controlling Na^+ and water excretion. If this mechanism is disturbed there will be uncontrolled Na^+ and water retention, resulting in hypertension. Hypertension is defined by the World Health Organization (WHO) as a sustained BP of 140/90 mmHg or above.

Essential hypertension

This accounts for about 95% of all cases of hypertension and the cause is unknown. Initially, there is an increase in cardiac output as a result of sympathetic overactivity. In the later stages the increase in BP is maintained by an increase in the TPR, but cardiac output is normal. Hypertensive changes seen in the kidney include:

- Arteriosclerosis of the major renal arteries (renal artery stenosis).
- Hyalinization of the small vessels with intimal thickening.

This can lead to chronic renal damage (hypertensive nephrosclerosis) and a reduction in the size of the kidneys.

Malignant or 'accelerated' hypertension is a rare and rapidly progressing form of severe hypertension. It is characterized by fibrinoid necrosis of the blood vessel walls, and ischaemic damage to the brain and kidney. This can lead to acute renal failure or heart failure, requiring urgent treatment.

Secondary hypertension

This is caused by renal (80%) and endocrine diseases, and occasionally drugs (ciclosporin A).

Renal mechanisms causing hypertension include:

- Impaired sodium and water excretion, increasing blood volume.
- Stimulation of renin release.

Renal causes of hypertension are:
- Renal artery stenosis (renovascular hypertension).
- Intrinsic renal disease (renal hypertension).
- Primary hyperaldosteronism (causing renal Na^+ retention and K^+ excretion).
- Excess renin production (e.g. renal tumour).

Renal artery stenosis

This accounts for 25% of renal-induced hypertension cases. There are two types:
- Atherosclerosis: common.
- Fibromuscular dysplasia: rare (seen in young women) (see Fig. 4.11).

Narrowing of the renal vessels reduces the pressure in the afferent arterioles, which stimulates the juxtaglomerular apparatus to secrete renin. This increases plasma angiotensin II, which causes vasoconstriction and aldosterone release. Aldosterone promotes Na$^+$ and therefore fluid retention (this increases BP), and increases K$^+$ secretion.

Treatment involves:
- Transluminal angioplasty (to dilate the stenotic region), supplemented with stenting.
- Reconstructive vascular surgery.
- Nephrectomy.

Up to 50% of the patients are cured or improved following treatment.

Intrinsic renal diseases

These account for 75% of renal induced hypertension and include chronic glomerulonephritis (GN), chronic pyelonephritis and polycystic kidney disease.

Patients with primary glomerular disease present with hypertension—which is more severe—earlier than patients with renal interstitial disease.

Endocrine causes

The endocrine causes are:
- Cushing's syndrome.
- Oestrogen (i.e. the contraceptive pill and pregnancy).
- Phaeochromocytoma (rare).
- Primary hyperaldosteronism (Conn's syndrome).

Primary hyperaldosteronism is a rare condition in which there is chronic excessive secretion of aldosterone because of an adrenal cortical adenoma (Fig. 4.15). Patients present with hypertension and hypokalaemia. The reason why hypertension develops is unknown, because the increase in ECF volume is small. Diagnosis is made with a triad of:
- Hypokalaemia.
- Increased aldosterone.
- Decreased renin.

Treatment is by surgical removal of the adenoma, with a cure rate of 60%.

Management of hypertension

It is difficult to detect and treat hypertension because it is often asymptomatic, and many patients are reluctant to take medication if they feel well. It is very important to exclude an underlying cause of hypertension.

Hypertension is an important risk factor for strokes, cardiac failure, myocardial infarction and renal failure. Effective treatment will improve the prognosis for each of these conditions.

Lifestyle changes include:
- Weight reduction.
- Reduced alcohol intake.
- Salt restriction.
- Regular exercise.
- Stop smoking.

Drug treatment of hypertension involves:
- Diuretics (i.e. loop diuretics and thiazide diuretics—see p. 90).
- Angiotensin-converting enzyme (ACE) inhibitors.
- β-blockers.
- Vasodilators (i.e. Ca^{2+} channel blockers).

Fig. 4.15 Mechanism by which an adrenal tumour (Conn's syndrome) causes secondary hypertension.

Angiotensin-converting enzyme (ACE) inhibitors

These inhibit ACE, and so block formation of angiotensin II. Angiotensin II is a potent vasoconstrictor and promotes sodium reabsorption in the tubule. This system is stimulated by:

- Renal arteriolar pressure.
- Sympathetic stimulation.
- Reduced delivery of sodium to the distal tubule (Fig. 4.16).

ACE inhibitors (e.g. captopril, enalapril) lower BP by:

- Reducing TPR.
- Inhibiting the local (tissue) renin–angiotensin system.

ACE inhibitors also reduce proteinuria and delay the progress of renal disease in diabetic patients. They are also used to treat CCF.

The side-effects of ACE inhibitors include:

- Persistent dry cough.
- Allergic reactions or rashes.
- Dose-related proteinuria.
- Changes in the sensation of taste.
- Severe hypotension especially in patients who are hypovolaemic.
- Acute renal failure in patients with renal artery stenosis (check this before giving ACE inhibitors).
- Hyperkalaemia.

ACE inhibitors are contraindicated in the final two trimesters of pregnancy because of the risk of:

- Developmental abnormalities in the fetal kidney.
- Oligohydramnios (reduced amniotic fluid).
- Neonatal hypotension and anuria.

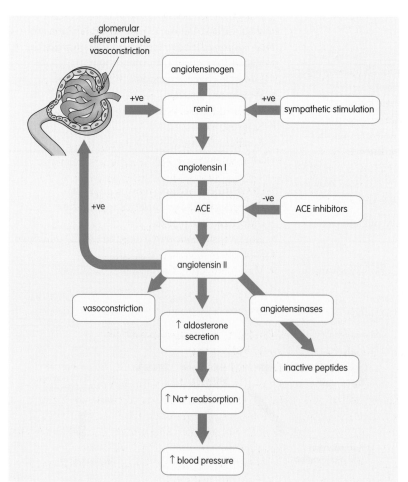

Fig. 4.16 Effects of ACE (angiotensin-converting enzyme) inhibitors. +ve, positive feedback; –ve, negative feedback.

Side-effects of the ACE inhibitor captopril:
- **C**ough.
- **A**llergic reaction.
- **P**roteinuria.
- **T**aste changes.
- Hyp**O**tension.
- **P**regnancy—fetal renal failure.
- **R**ash.
- Makes you **ILL**!

Hepatorenal syndrome

Patients with liver disease can have a reduced urine flow (oliguria). This is especially so in patients with portal hypertension and ascites. Portal hypertension results from an increase in resistance to blood flow from the gut and spleen, resulting in venous congestion due to nitric oxide release. This stimulates renin release. As there appears to be a fall in arterial blood volume, Na^+ and water are retained. As a result of increased resistance in the liver caused by hepatic cirrhosis, hydrostatic pressure in the portal vein increases. This causes fluid to accumulate in the peritoneal cavity (ascites) as fluid is forced out of the interstitial capillaries. This further reduces the circulating blood volume, which again stimulates renin release. Thus, a positive feedback loop promoting hypertension is set up.

Liver disease can also impair albumin synthesis. This decreases the oncotic (colloid osmotic) pressure in the capillaries, favouring fluid movement out and worsening the ascites. Circulating blood volume is further reduced.

Nephrotic syndrome

This is a chronic condition characterized by:
- Proteinuria (>3g/24h): sufficient to cause:
- Hypoalbuminaemia (serum albumin < 25g/L): sufficient to cause oedema and secondary hypercholesterolaemia.

There is increased permeability of the glomerular filter to albumin as a result of glomerular basement membrane damage and increase in pore size. In an adult a loss of more than 3–5g of albumin per day can cause hypoalbuminaemia, but some patients can have nephrotic-range proteinuria without being overtly nephrotic, because the rate of albumin synthesis compensates for the albumin loss. A limited amount of filtered protein can be reabsorbed by endocytosis,

but if this is exceeded, protein is lost in the urine. The albumin content within the capillary helps maintain the colloid osmotic pressure. If this decreases, less fluid moves back into the capillaries, causing oedema in the peripheral tissues. The decreased circulating volume stimulates the renin–angiotensin–aldosterone sytem, leading to further sodium and water retention, and further oedema.

Treatment

Management includes:
- Blood pressure control.
- Reduction of proteinuria, using ACE inhibitors and non-steroidal anti-inflammatory drugs (NSAIDs).
- Control of hyperlipidaemia.
- Anticoagulation if hypercoagulable (risk of thrombosis increases as albumin decreases).
- Treatment of underlying causes, e.g. in minimal change disease. High-dose corticosteroid therapy will treat protein leakage in 90% of children; the response is much lower in adults.

Complications of nephrotic syndrome include:
- Hypercoagulable state: increases risk of deep vein thrombosis (DVT), pulmonary embolus (PE) and renal vein thrombosis.
- Hyperlipidaemia: increases risk of vascular disease and ischaemic heart disease.
- Immunosuppression: increases risk of infection.

A major complication of nephrotic syndrome is renal vein thrombosis, which should be suspected if proteinuria increases or renal function deteriorates. Diagnosis is by ultrasound, and treatment involves anticoagulation.

Interventions in renal disease

Medical management of renal disease
Diuretics

Diuretics increase the volume of urine produced by increasing renal sodium excretion (natriuresis), which is followed passively by water. Each type of diuretic has specific actions on the normal physiology of a particular segment (Fig. 4.17):
- Act on the membrane transport proteins found on the luminal surface.

key	

1 proximal tubule
• osmotic diuresis
  (e.g. mannitol)
• carbonic anhydrase inhibitor
  (e.g. acetazolamide)
	3 distal tubule
	• K⁺-sparing diuretic
	  (e.g. amiloride)
	• thiazides

2 ascending loop of Henle
• loop diuretics
  (e.g. furosemide)
	4 collecting duct
	• K⁺-sparing diuretics
	  (e.g. spironolactone)

Fig. 4.17 Sites of diuretic action.

- Interfere with hormone receptors.
- Inhibit enzyme activity.

Osmotic diuretics

Osmotic diuresis can be induced by an inert substance that is not reabsorbed in the tubule. The proximal tubule and the descending limb of the loop of Henle allow free movement of water molecules. If an agent such as mannitol is introduced into the tubular fluid, it is not absorbed and thus reduces water reabsorption. There is increased urine flow through the nephrons resulting in reduced sodium reabsorption.

Osmotic diuretics are used to:
- Increase urine volume when renal haemodynamics are compromised, and thus prevent anuria.
- Reduce intracranial pressures in neurological conditions.
- Reduce intraocular pressures before ophthalmic surgery.

Excessive use of osmotic diuretics without adequate fluid replacement can cause dehydration and hypernatraemia.

Loop diuretics

These are the most powerful diuretics, causing up to 20% of filtered Na^+ to be excreted. They inhibit sodium transport out of the thick ascending limb of the loop of Henle into the medullary interstitium. Examples include furosemide (frusemide) and bumetanide. Loop diuretics (e.g. frusemide) act by inhibiting the $Na^+/K^+/2Cl^-$ cotransporter on the luminal membrane of the cells. This inhibits Na^+ reabsorption, thereby diluting the osmotic gradient in the medulla. This results in increased Na^+ and water excretion. Positive lumen potential falls as cations are retained, causing an increase in Ca^{2+} and Mg^{2+} excretion. As a higher $[Na^+]$ reaches the distal tubule, there is increased K^+ secretion, so loop diuretics can be used to reduce total body K^+.

Loop diuretics are used for:
- Acute pulmonary and peripheral oedema.
- To reduce end-diastolic ventricular filling pressure.
- Pulmonary congestion.
- Acute hypercalcaemia.
- Hypertension.
- Nephrotic syndrome.
- Acute renal failure (increases urine output and K^+ excretion).

The side-effects of loop diuretics include:
- Hypokalaemic metabolic alkalosis.
- Hypovolaemia and hypotension.
- Hyperuricaemia (can precipitate attacks of gout).
- Hypomagnesaemia.
- Ototoxicity (dose-related reversible auditory loss).
- Allergic reactions.

Thiazide diuretics

These reduce active Na^+ reabsorption in the early distal tubule by inhibiting the Na^+/Cl^- cotransporter. As there is more reabsorption of Na^+ in the loop of

Henle, the loop diuretics are more potent than thiazide diuretics. Thiazides help reduce peripheral vascular resistance, and consequently are used to manage hypertension. They are also used in CCF and nephrogenic diabetes insipidus.

Renal-related side-effects of thiazide diuretics include:
- Hypokalaemic metabolic alkalosis.
- Hyperglycaemia.
- Hyperlipidaemia.
- Hyperuricaemia.
- Hypercalcaemia.
- Hyponatraemia.

Side-effects unrelated to renal actions include hypercholesterolaemia, reversible male impotence and allergic reactions (rare).

Side-effects of thiazide diuretics: HyperGLUC (hyper glucose, lipid, uric acid and calcium).

Potassium-sparing diuretics
These diuretics are K^+-sparing and act:
- In the collecting ducts (e.g. spironolactone).
- By inhibiting the uptake of Na^+ in the cells of the distal nephron (e.g. amiloride and triamterene).

Aldosterone is a mineralocorticoid that increases the activity of the Na^+/K^+ ATPase, potassium and sodium channels, resulting in Na^+ absorption and K^+ secretion.

Spironolactone (a mineralocorticoid analogue) competes with aldosterone for the receptor site. This reduces sodium reabsorption in the distal nephron and decreases K^+ secretion (potassium-sparing activity).

Potassium-sparing diuretics are used if there is mineralocorticoid excess such as primary aldosteronism (Conn's syndrome) or ectopic ACTH production. They are also used in secondary aldosteronism where salt and water retention have occurred (e.g. CCF, nephrotic syndrome, liver disease and hypovolaemia). They are fairly weak, often used with loop diuretics or thiazides to prevent K^+ loss.

The side-effects include:
- Hyperkalaemia: this results from an increase in H^+—and therefore K^+—retention as Na^+ absorption falls and ranges from mild to life-threatening.

- Endocrine effects with spironolactone (e.g. gynaecomastia).

Potassium-sparing diuretics are contraindicated in patients with chronic renal insufficiency.

Carbonic anhydrase (CA) inhibitors
CA is found in many places in the nephron but primarily on the brush border of the luminal membrane of the proximal tubule cells. CA catalyses the dehydration of H_2CO_3:

$$H^+ + HCO_3^- \leftrightarrow H_2CO_3 \leftrightarrow H_2O + CO_2$$

This reaction is driven by H^+ secretion into the lumen, by cotransport with Na^+. Once in the cell, H_2CO_3 is reformed under the influence of intracellular CA, the HCO_3^- ions are reabsorbed, and H^+ is secreted back into the lumen (see Fig. 2.24).

CA inhibitors interfere with the action of carbonic anhydrase and inhibit HCO_3^- reabsorption. The presence of HCO_3^- in the lumen reduces Na^+ reabsorption, which continues into the distal nephron where it enhances K^+ secretion.

CA inhibitors such as acetazolamide are weak diuretics, which cause the excretion of only about 5–10% of the filtered Na^+ and water. Their main clinical use is to treat acute and chronic glaucoma by reducing intraocular pressure (the production of aqueous humour in the eye involves secretion of HCO_3^- by the ciliary body in a process similar to that in the proximal tubule).

The side-effects of CA inhibitors include:
- Metabolic acidosis.
- Renal stones.
- Renal K^+ wasting.
- Nervous system effects—paraesthesia and drowsiness.

CA inhibitors should be avoided in patients with liver disease or advanced chronic renal failure.

A summary of the main classes of diuretic is shown in Fig. 4.18.

Dialysis and haemofiltration
Dialysis imitates the kidney by temporarily removing waste products and excess fluids that accumulate in renal failure. It is used to treat renal failure in patients with acute or chronic renal failure. Dialysis is indicated when there is:
- Creatinine clearance <5ml/min.
- GFR <5%.
- Blood urea >30mmol/L.

Summary of the three main classes of diuretic			
Class	Loop diuretics	Thiazide diuretics	K+-sparing diuretics
diuretic capability	+++	++	+
site of action	thick ascending loop of Henle	distal tubule	collecting tubule
mechanism of action	inhibit Na+/K+/2Cl− cotransporter, and thus increase Na+ and K+ loss	inhibit the Na+/Cl− cotransporter (K+ loss, Ca2+ loss)	block Na+ channels and thus antagonize aldosterone receptors
side-effects	hypokalaemia; metabolic acidosis; hypovolaemia	hypokalaemia; metabolic alkalosis	hyperkalaemia
example	furosemide (frusemide)	bendroflumethiazide (bendrofluazide)	spironolactone; amiloride

Fig. 4.18 Summary of the three main classes of diuretics.

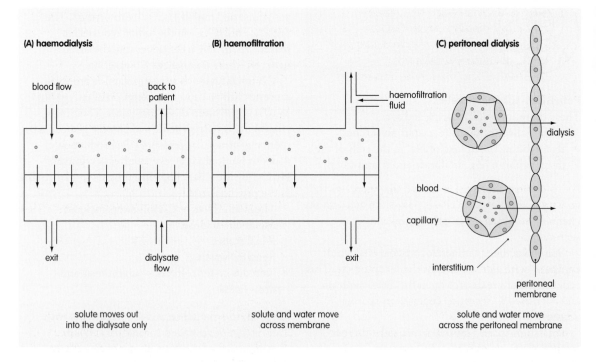

Fig. 4.19 Comparison of the three different methods of dialysis. (A) haemodialysis; (B) haemofiltration and (C) peritoneal dialysis (adapted from O'Callaghan CA, Bremmer BM 2001 The kidney at a glance. Blackwell Science, p 96, 98).

- Hyperkalaemia.
- Acidosis.
- Fluid overload.

A semi-permeable membrane acts as a filter, with a dialysate solution to regulate the fluid and electrolytes in the blood. There are three forms of dialysis: haemodialysis, haemofiltration and continuous ambulatory peritoneal dialysis (Fig. 4.19). At best, it provides an equivalent average clearance of approximately 10mL/min (normal GFR, 125mL/min).

Haemodialysis

This involves pumping the blood through an artificial kidney, called a dialysis machine. Blood flows on one side of a semi-permeable membrane, with dialysis fluid being passed in the opposite direction on the other side. Typically, blood flows at 300mL/min and the dialysate fluid flows at 500mL/min. Dialysis occurs across the semi-permeable membrane removing toxins from the blood down a concentration gradient.

Several synthetic semi-permeable membranes are available, with different permeability characteristics. The dialysate is made of purified water with a solute composition similar to plasma, but without any of the waste products, so solutes move along their concentration gradient out of the blood.

Access to the circulation is gained by an arteriovenous (AV) fistula, which is constructed surgically, usually by joining the radial artery and cephalic vein. The venous system 'arterialises' and the high blood flows required for dialysis can be obtained by 'needling' the venous system. Complications of the AV fistula include infection and thrombosis.

Dialysis 'dose' can be adjusted by altering the blood flow, the area of the semi-permeable membrane, or the duration of treatment. On average, patients require approximately 4h of treatment three times a week.

Complications of haemodialysis include:
- Hypotension.
- Infection.
- Haemolysis.
- Air embolism.
- Reactions to dialysis membrane.

Haemofiltration

This involves filtering blood across a semi-permeable membrane allowing removal of small molecules. The fluid is replaced with that of the appropriate biochemical composition. The replacement fluid is commonly buffered by lactate. Haemofiltration is used in acute renal failure (ARF) and chronic renal failure (CRF). It causes smaller fluid shifts and therefore less hypotension than haemodialysis.

Both haemodialysis and haemofiltration can be used continuously in ARF to ensure slow continuous correction of the fluid and electrolyte balance, especially in patients with haemodynamic instability.

Continuous ambulatory peritoneal dialysis (CAPD)

This procedure uses the peritoneal membrane as the semi-permeable membrane. Unlike haemodialysis, peritoneal dialysis does not require an AV fistula for circulatory access. Instead, it requires the insertion of a permanent 'Tenchkoff' catheter through the anterior abdominal wall into the peritoneal cavity. Dialysate solution is introduced into the peritoneum and exchanged regularly for fresh fluid—up to five times a day is necessary to maintain the efficiency of dialysis. Waste products pass into the dialysate along their concentration gradients and water is removed by osmosis. Dialysis solutions with high osmolarity will remove more water. Dextrose is commonly used to induce osmosis, but is gradually absorbed by the patient. Newer, non-absorbable, osmotic agents are now available (e.g. glucose polymer). CAPD is used in the maintenance dialysis of end-stage renal failure, but technique survival declines to 50% after 5 years due to loss of peritoneal membrane function.

Complications of peritoneal dialysis include:
- Peritonitis (50% is caused by *Staphylococcus epidermidis*). Treatment is with intraperitoneal or intravenous antibiotics.
- Mechanical problems with fluid drainage.
- Infections or blockage around the site of the catheter.

Other complications include constipation, pleural effusions and sclerosing peritonitis (rare but serious).

Contraindications to CAPD are:
- Peritoneal adhesions as a result of peritonitis.
- Abdominal hernia.
- Colostomy.

Dialysis is essential in patients presenting with hyperkalaemia, acidosis, pulmonary oedema and uraemic complications.

Renal transplantation

This is the most successful organ transplant and is the ideal treatment for end-stage irreversible renal failure. It restores near-normal renal function and improves quality of life. The kidney comes from a cadaver or a close living relative and is usually placed in the iliac fossa. The renal vessels from the donated kidney are anastomosed onto the iliac blood vessels

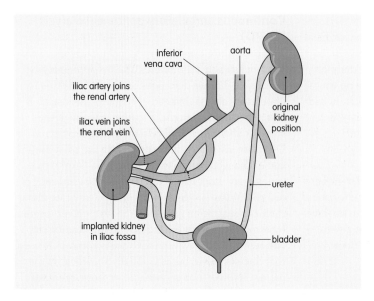

Fig. 4.20 Implantation of a transplanted kidney.

Labels in figure:
- inferior vena cava
- aorta
- iliac artery joins the renal artery
- original kidney position
- iliac vein joins the renal vein
- ureter
- implanted kidney in iliac fossa
- bladder

of the recipient and the ureter is inserted into the bladder (Fig. 4.20). Success depends upon:

- ABO group.
- Matching the donor and the recipient for human leucocyte antigen (HLA) types.
- Preoperative blood transfusion.
- Immunosuppressive treatment.

Short-term complications include:

- Acute rejection (within 3 months).
- Operative failure.

Rejection is reduced by immunosuppression therapy, which is started after the transplant and continued indefinitely. However, patients are at risk of opportunistic infection (e.g. with cytomegalovirus).

Long-term complications include:

- Infection.
- Recurrence of original disease.
- Obstruction at the ureteric anastomoses.
- Malignancy, especially lymphomas.

Currently, the 1-year graft survival rate is 80% for cadaveric transplants and 90% for live donor transplants.

- Compare and contrast unilateral and bilateral renal agenesis. Explain what causes renal agenesis.
- Name the genes that have been identified in adult polycystic kidney disease. Discuss how the prognosis in adult polycystic kidney disease differs from that in childhood polycystic kidney disease.
- Outline the system used to classify glomerular disease.
- Discuss the five main clinical syndromes associated with the clinical manifestations of glomerular disease, giving clinical examples.
- Explain how nephritic syndrome (i.e. acute nephritis) differs from nephrotic syndrome.
- Describe the systemic manifestations of HSP.
- Outline the causes of ATN.
- Discuss the incidence, presentation and diagnosis of UTIs.
- For acute and chronic pyelonephritis, discuss the aetiology, prediposing factors, appearance of the kidney and histology.
- Outline the changes seen in the renal vasculature in hypertension. Describe the two main types of hypertension.
- Describe the histological changes and management of renal artery stenosis.
- Explain the abbreviation HUS. Describe the major differences between the two main types.
- Discuss renal cell carcinoma, noting its incidence, the age group affected, predisposing factors, presentation and morphology.
- Describe a Wilms' tumour and clarify which age group it affects.
- Explain the compensatory mechanisms that come into effect in CCF.
- Outline the different types of shock and their effects on renal physiology.
- Describe which immune disorders affect the kidney.
- Discuss the site and mechanism of action, uses and side-effects for each of the different diuretics.
- Outline the use of ACE inhibitors in the treatment of hypertension, indicating their mechanisms of action and side-effects.
- Explain how the three types of dialysis differ.

5. The Lower Urinary Tract

Organization of the lower urinary tract

Macroscopic organization
Overview
Urine formed in the kidneys collects in the renal pelvis and then passes down the lower urinary tract (ureters, bladder and urethra) before exiting the body. The bladder stores the urine, which is ejected intermittently from the body under voluntary control.

Ureters
The ureters are hollow muscular tubes 25–30cm long, which begin as funnel-shaped tubes at the renal pelvis. They run retroperitoneally over the posterior abdominal wall in front of the external iliac artery down to the pelvic brim (similar course in the female). Figures 5.1 and 5.2 show the course of the ureters through the pelvis in a man and woman, respectively. As urine collects in the renal pelvis, the pelvis dilates. Action potentials in the pacemaker cells of the renal pelvis are set up, stimulating peristaltic contractions in the ureters that propel the urine (Fig. 5.3).

The ureters are divided into regions related to their anatomical course: renal pelvis, abdominal, pelvic and intramural regions (Fig. 5.4). This influences the source of blood supply to each region of the ureter—renal, lumbar segmental, gonadal, common iliac, internal iliac and superior vesical arteries, with corresponding venous drainage.

The ureters are innervated by both sympathetic and parasympathetic nerves. Sensory nerves are from T11–L2 and S2–4, but the motor supply to the muscular wall is unclear. As shown in Fig. 5.4 there are constrictions in the ureters. Stones can get stuck at these constrictions and produce acute colicky pain, which is referred to the skin of T11–L2. Therefore, pain starts in the loin and radiates to the scrotum and penis (men) or to the labium majus (women).

Lymphatic drainage is to the para-aortic lymph nodes.

Reflux of urine from the bladder back into the ureter is prevented by a valvular mechanism at the vesicoureteric junction.

Urinary bladder
The ureters enter the base of the bladder, which is partially covered by peritoneum.
- When empty, it lies in the pelvis and rests on the symphysis pubis and floor of the pelvis.
- When filled, it enlarges into the abdominal cavity.

The neck of the bladder is relatively immobile and fixed by the puboprostatic and lateral vesical ligament. Figure 5.5 shows the internal and external aspects of the male bladder and Fig. 5.2 shows the urinary bladder in the female. The blood supply to the bladder is from the superior and inferior vesical branches of the internal iliac artery. It is drained by the vesical plexus and by the prostatic venous plexus in the male, which then drain into the internal iliac vein. Lymphatic drainage is also along the vesical blood vessels to the internal iliac nodes, then the para-aortic nodes.

Interior of the bladder
The wall is yellow with rugae (folds) allowing expansion with little increase in internal pressure. The base is the trigone, which is a triangular reddish region bounded by the ureteric openings into the bladder and the internal urethral meatus (see Fig. 5.5). This area is less mobile and less distensible than the rest of the bladder. It is more sensitive to painful stimuli.

The bladder is lined by smooth muscle, known as the detrusor muscle, which, like the ureter, is arranged in spiral, long and circular bundles. Smooth muscle bundles surround the bladder neck to form the internal urethral sphincter, which is under involuntary control. Slightly further along the urethra there is a skeletal muscle sphincter—the external urethral sphincter. This is under voluntary control.

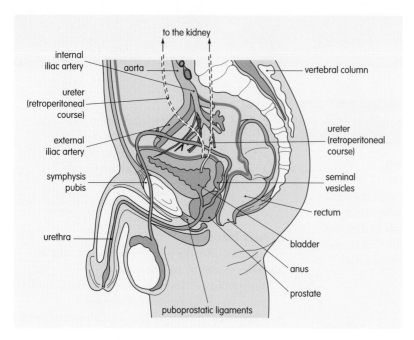

Fig. 5.1 Anatomy of the male lower urinary tract.

- internal iliac artery
- aorta
- to the kidney
- vertebral column
- ureter (retroperitoneal course)
- external iliac artery
- ureter (retroperitoneal course)
- symphysis pubis
- seminal vesicles
- rectum
- urethra
- bladder
- anus
- prostate
- puboprostatic ligaments

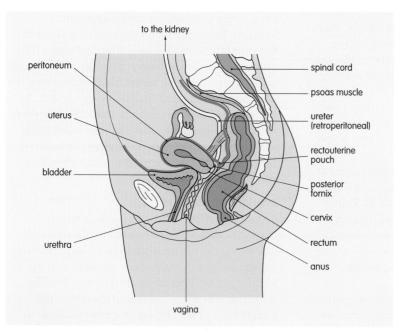

Fig. 5.2 Anatomy of the female lower urinary tract.

- to the kidney
- peritoneum
- spinal cord
- psoas muscle
- uterus
- ureter (retroperitoneal)
- rectouterine pouch
- bladder
- posterior fornix
- cervix
- urethra
- rectum
- anus
- vagina

- The internal urethral sphincter is not under voluntary control, and thus contracts reflexly.
- The external urethral sphincter is under voluntary control.

Bladder innervation (Fig. 5.6) is both:
- **Sensory:** gives sensation (awareness) of a full bladder and also pain from disease. The impulses are suppressed if the bladder is empty.
- **Motor:** parasympathetic activity stimulates the detrusor muscle, so the bladder contracts. It also inhibits the external urethral sphincter, which relaxes to allow micturition. Sympathetic activity

Fig. 5.3 Mechanism of ureteric peristalsis.

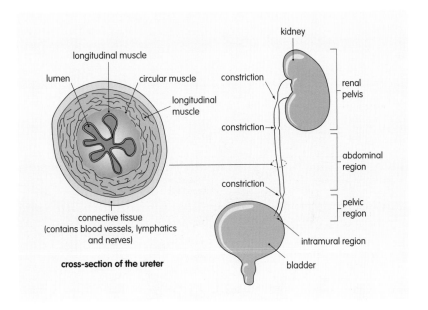

Fig. 5.4 Regions of the ureter and cross-sectional view, highlighting the normal points of reduced diameter at which stones commonly lodge.

inhibits the detrusor muscle, so the bladder relaxes, and stimulates the urethral sphincter (this contracts). Both these actions prevent micturition.

Male urethra

The male urethra (Fig. 5.7) is longer than the female urethra (male = 20 cm, female = 4 cm). It runs through the neck of bladder, the prostate gland, the floor of pelvis and the perineal membrane to the penis and external urethral orifice at the tip of the glans penis. It has three parts:

1. Prostatic urethra: surrounded by prostate tissue.
2. Membranous urethra: the shortest region, with sphincter activity.
3. Spongy urethra: surrounded by penile tissue.

It is innervated by the prostatic plexus and lymphatic drainage is to the internal iliac and deep inguinal nodes.

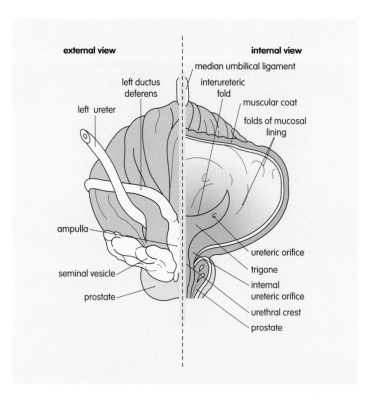

Fig. 5.5 Posterior and interior view of the male bladder.

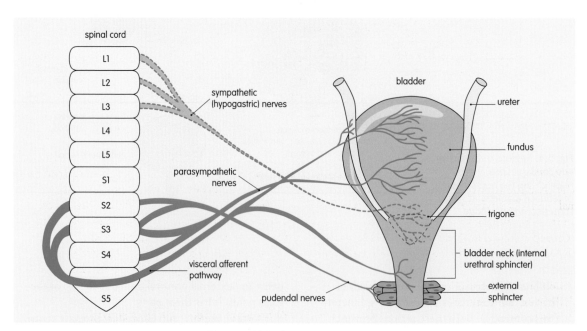

Fig. 5.6 Innervation of the bladder (from Koeppen BM, Stanton B 1996 Renal physiology, 2nd edn. Mosby Year Book).

Female urethra

This starts at the neck of the bladder and passes through the floor of the pelvis and perineal membrane to open into the vestibule just anterior to the opening of the vagina. It is 4 cm in length and is firmly attached to the anterior wall of the vagina. Lymphatics drain to the internal and external iliac lymph nodes.

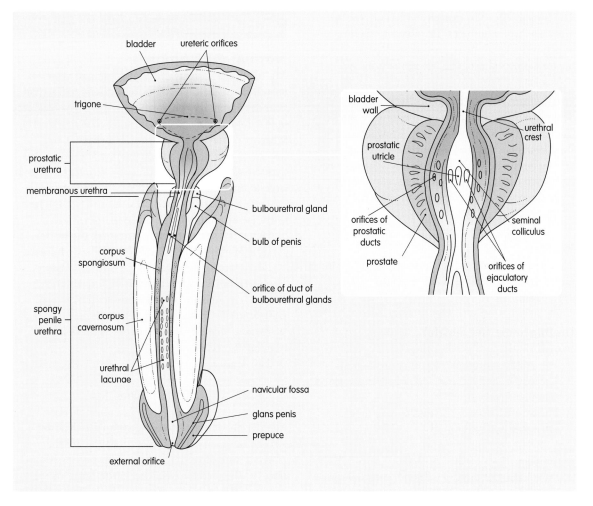

Fig. 5.7 The male urethra.

Prostate

This is a gland lying below the bladder in the male and surrounding the proximal part of the urethra ('prostatic urethra'). It measures $4 \times 3 \times 2$ cm and is conical in shape. It is connected to the bladder by connective tissue stroma and has three parts:

1. Left lateral lobe.
2. Right lateral lobe.
3. Middle lobe.

The prostate has a connective tissue capsule, which is surrounded by a thick sheath from the pelvic fascia. It is influenced by sex hormones resulting in growth during puberty. From the 4th decade onwards, it hypertrophies and nodules of hyperplastic glandular and connective tissue form. As the prostate surrounds the urethra, any enlargement can narrow the urethra and obstruct urine flow.

The prostate is supplied by the inferior vesical artery and blood drains via the prostatic plexus to the vesical plexus and internal iliac vein. Lymphatics drain to the internal iliac and sacral nodes. The prostatic plexus innervates the prostate.

Microstructure of the distal urinary tract
Ureters

The muscular layers are made of smooth muscle (see Fig. 5.4) arranged in layers:

- A longitudinal layer just outside the lumen.
- A middle circular layer.
- Another longitudinal layer.

The lumen is lined by urinary epithelium (also known as urothelium or transitional epithelium), which is folded in the relaxed state allowing the ureter to dilate during the passage of urine.

Urothelium (transitional epithelium)
The plasma membranes of urothelium are thicker than other cell membranes, preventing interstitial fluid from entering the concentrated urine. Urothelium is impermeable to urine. The cells have highly interdigitating cell junctions, allowing the epithelium to stretch without damaging the surfaces of the cells.

Bladder
This is similar to that of the lower third of the ureter, with smooth muscle walls and transitional epithelium.

Urethra (male and female)
In males:
- The prostatic urethra is lined by urothelium.
- The rest is lined by stratified or pseudostratified columnar epithelium.
- The external opening is lined by stratified squamous epithelium.

In females:
- Proximally, the urethra is lined by urothelium.
- Distally and at the external opening, the urethra is lined by stratified squamous epithelium.

Prostate
The prostate contains a central zone of mucosal glands originating prenatally from the endoderm. These drain directly into the urethra. There is also a peripheral zone of mucosal glands, derived from the mesoderm, which drains into the ducts that enter the urethral sinus. Prostatic glandular epithelium can vary from inactive low cuboidal cells to active pseudostratified columnar cells, depending on the degree of androgen stimulation from the testes. The glands secrete 75% of seminal fluid, which is thin, milky and rich in citric acid and hydrolytic enzymes (e.g. fibrinolysin). This prostatic secretion liquefies coagulated semen after deposition in the female genital tract. The prostate is covered by a stroma and capsule made of dense fibroelastic connective tissue with a smooth muscle component.

Micturition

Normal micturition
Micturition is the intermittent voiding of urine stored in the bladder. It is an autonomic reflex that is under voluntary control. The inside of the bladder wall is folded and can expand and accommodate fluid with little increase in pressure. However, it can accommodate only a certain volume of fluid before an increase in intravesical pressure occurs, causing an urge to micturate. Figure 5.8 shows a normal cystometrogram in which pressure rise is compared with rise in volume in the bladder.

Figure 5.6 shows the innervation of the bladder. In infants, micturition is a local spinal reflex where the bladder empties upon reaching a critical pressure. However, in adults this reflex is under voluntary control, so can be inhibited or initiated by higher centres in the brain. During micturition:
- Perineal muscles and the external urethral sphincter relax.
- The detrusor muscle contracts (parasympathetic activity).
- Urine flows out of the bladder.

Bladder distension with urine stimulates bladder stretch receptors, which, in turn, stimulate the afferent limb of voiding reflex and parasympathetic fibres of the bladder, resulting in the desire to urinate. Higher-centre stimulation of the pudendal

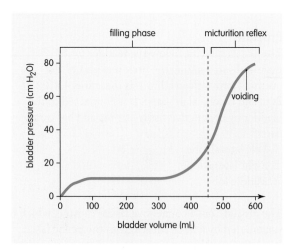

Fig. 5.8 Normal cystometrogram showing the rise in pressure associated with increasing bladder volume.

nerves keeps the external sphincter closed until it is appropriate to urinate. Figure 5.9 illustrates the voluntary control of micturition.

Abnormal micturition
Neurological lesions
Urinary continence is affected by various neurological lesions along the micturition pathway, as summarized in Fig. 5.10.

Lesion in the superior frontal gyrus
This can be the result of a stroke, and leads to:
- Reduced desire to urinate.
- Difficulty stopping micturition once started.

Lesion of afferent nerves from the bladder
A lesion of afferent nerves from the bladder (e.g. caused by disease of the dorsal roots such as tabes dorsalis) prevents reflex contractions of the bladder, so the bladder becomes distended, thin walled and hypotonic.

Lesion of both afferent and efferent nerves
A lesion of both afferent and efferent nerves (e.g. because of a tumour of the cauda equina or filum terminale) results in:
- Initially: bladder flaccidity and distension.
- Later: bladder hyperactivity with dribbling.

This leads to a shrunken bladder with a hypertrophied bladder wall.

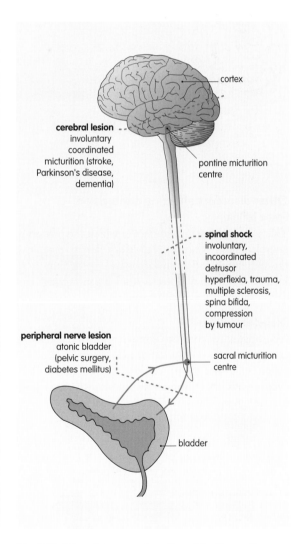

Fig. 5.9 Voluntary control of micturition.

Fig. 5.10 Sites of damage along the micturition pathway.

Spinal cord lesion

A lesion to the spinal cord (e.g. spinal shock sustained following trauma) results in:

- Initially: overflow incontinence, because of a flaccid and unresponsive bladder, which results in overfill and dribbling. This is spinal shock.
- After shock has passed: the voiding reflex returns, but with no control from higher centres, so the patient has no voluntary control over voiding.
- Occasionally: hyperactive voiding might be seen.
- Eventually: bladder capacity falls and the wall hypertrophies—spastic neurogenic bladder.

Spinal cord injuries lead to reflex micturition, as is seen in infants. This occurs because, like infants, patients with spinal cord lesions cannot synchronize detrusor muscle contractions with sphincter relaxation.

Other disorders affecting micturition

Spina bifida

This is a developmental defect in which the posterior neural arches of the spine fail to develop, so part of the spinal cord and its coverings are exposed. It forms a spectrum of defects, resulting in varying degrees of bladder dysfunction.

Diabetes mellitus

Neuropathy is a common complication of diabetes. It can result in a loss of sensation, so there is no desire to micturate and the patient voids infrequently. This eventually leads to bladder distension, with overflow incontinence. The presence of residual urine increases the risk of infection.

Multiple sclerosis

This is demyelination of white matter. The bladder symptoms that develop depend on the level at which demyelination occurs.

Pelvic surgery

The nerve supply to the bladder can be injured during surgery, resulting in postoperative urinary retention. This is usually transient.

Congenital abnormalities of the urinary tract

Ureteric abnormalities

These occur in 2–5% of the population. They are frequently bilateral and have usually no clinical relevance. Occasionally, however, they might be associated with an obstruction of urine flow.

Double and bifid ureters

The ureters along with the calyces and collecting ducts are formed from an outgrowth of the mesonephric (Wolffian) duct called the ureteric bud. Early splitting of the ureteric bud or the development of two buds results in the development of double (bifid) ureters (Fig. 5.11). The duplication can be:

- Partial: the two ureters meet before entering the bladder together.
- Complete: the two ureters enter the bladder separately. The upper pole ureter enters the bladder lower and more medially than the lower ureter (see Fig. 5.11).

It is often associated with double renal pelvises with their own renal parenchyma. Renal function is rarely affected. There is a strong predisposition to infection. Urine can reflux from the bladder, especially through the upper pole ureter. Treatment involves excision of the refluxing ureter (usually the upper one).

Ureteropelvic junction obstruction

This often presents in infancy, although milder forms might not present until later in adult life or be found in asymptomatic patients at post-mortem. It is more common in males and in the left ureter. It is bilateral in 20% of cases, and might present as a mass in the flank or pain after drinking. It is thought to result from abnormal smooth muscle organization at the ureteropelvic junction. It can be accompanied by renal agenesis of the opposite kidney; the reason for this is unknown. As a result of the back pressure from the obstruction, the pelvicalyceal system (Fig. 5.12) dilates. If the pressure is transmitted up to the kidneys, the renal tissue atrophies. If bilateral, renal failure can result.

Diverticula

Diverticula are outpouchings of the ureteral wall; they are usually congenital. They are very common

Fig. 5.11 Partial and complete bifid ureter.

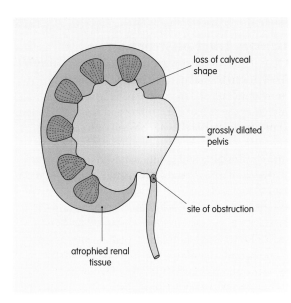

Fig. 5.12 Pelvicalyceal dilatation.

and create sites for the stasis of urine. This increases the risk of urine infection because the continuous flow of urine through the urinary tract is a protective mechanism against infection. Acquired diverticula

can develop if the pressure in the ureters increases (e.g. because of obstruction).

Hydroureter and megaloureter

Congenital hydroureters develop if there are neuromuscular defects in the wall of the ureter. They are sometimes associated with other congenital malformations in the genitourinary tract. There is dilatation, elongation and frequently tortuosity of the ureters. Acquired hydroureters develop in adults during pregnancy and lower urinary tract obstruction, where a persistently raised pressure within the bladder impairs ureter emptying. A ureter so dilated that transport of urine by peristalsis is compromised is known as a megaureter.

Bladder abnormalities
Diverticula

These are sac-like outpouchings through a weak point in the bladder wall. They can be either:
- Congenital: these develop in localized areas of defective muscle within the wall or because of urinary tract obstruction in fetal development. They are usually solitary lesions, most commonly occurring close to the ureterovesical junction.

105

- Acquired: these usually develop much later in life as a result of chronic urethral obstruction (e.g. prostatic hypertrophy). They are clinically significant and, characteristically, occur as multiple lesions.

In both cases, urine stasis increases the risk of bladder infection, leading to vesicoureteric reflux and eventual stone formation.

Exstrophy

Exstrophy of the bladder is a serious condition affecting the anterior wall of the bladder and anterior abdominal wall. It presents in infancy and is more common in males. The anterior wall of the bladder fails to develop, so the posterior wall lies exposed on the lower abdominal wall, causing squamous metaplasia of the mucosa. The mucosa is at high risk of infection. This disorder can vary in severity and can be associated with urethral and symphysis pubis defects. In the male there is epispadias, and in females a split clitoris. Surgical corrrection allows long-term survival of these infants. Despite treatment, there is an increased risk of adenocarcinomas of the bladder later in life, because of bladder extrusion.

Urethral abnormalities
Hypospadias

This is a spectrum of congenital abnormalities affecting 1 in 400 male infants. The urethra opens on the ventral surface of the penis, usually adjacent to the glans penis, but can open on the penile shaft or perineum. There is a ventral curvature to the penile shaft with a hooded prepuce. Surgical correction is carried out before the age of two to allow micturition with a straight stream.

Epispadias

The urethra opens on the dorsal surface of the penis. As with hypospadias, surgical correction is carried out before the age of two to allow micturition with a straight stream.

Urethral valves

Obstruction to urine flow can occur at the level of the posterior urethra in a boy due to the presence of mucosal folds or a membrane extending across the urethra (posterior urethral valve). The patient presents in early infancy with distended bladder,

dribbling, vomiting and failure to thrive. As a result of obstruction to urinary flow, male fetuses can have:
- Poor renal growth with reflux and dilated upper urinary tracts.
- Progressive bilateral hydronephrosis.
- Oligohydramnios (reduced volume of amniotic fluid).

Intrauterine intervention has no proven benefit and an early delivery is performed only if there are signs of rapidly progressing renal damage. Postnatal management includes:
- Prophylactic antibiotics from birth to prevent urinary tract infections (UTI).
- Ultrasound scans at birth and a few weeks later to assess the effect of the obstruction.

Surgical treatment is required in all cases. Any male child born with bilateral hydronephrosis must be investigated to exclude a posterior urethral valve.

Urinary tract obstruction and urolithiasis

Urinary tract obstruction

Obstruction in the urinary tract can occur at any level. It can be unilateral or bilateral, complete or incomplete, and of gradual or acute onset. It increases the risk of UTI, reflux and stone formation. If prolonged or unrelieved, obstruction can cause functional renal impairment and permanent renal atrophy. Imaging techniques involved in the diagnosis of urinary tract obstruction and its location (see Chapter 8) are:
- Ultrasound: identifies dilatation of the urinary tract.
- DTPA (diethylenetriamine penta-acetic acid) renography: confirms any functional obstruction.
- Intravenous urography (IVU): highlights anatomical and functional obstruction (cannot be used in patients with renal failure).
- Retrograde pyelography: can be necessary in some cases.

Careful imaging of the renal tract is essential to determine the site and cause of obstruction (see Chapter 8).

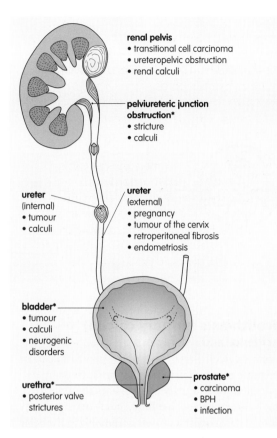

renal pelvis
• transitional cell carcinoma
• ureteropelvic obstruction
• renal calculi

pelviureteric junction obstruction*
• stricture
• calculi

ureter (internal)
• tumour
• calculi

ureter (external)
• pregnancy
• tumour of the cervix
• retroperitoneal fibrosis
• endometriosis

bladder*
• tumour
• calculi
• neurogenic disorders

urethra*
• posterior valve strictures

prostate*
• carcinoma
• BPH
• infection

Fig. 5.13 Sites of obstruction in the urinary tract (* indicate the most common sites of obstruction).

Causes of urinary obstruction

Figure 5.13 shows the sites of obstruction in the urinary tract. Obstruction is caused by a congenital defect or, more commonly, by a structural lesion.

Congenital abnormalities

These include the following neuromuscular defects:
• Urethral valves and strictures.
• Meatal strictures.
• Bladder neck obstruction.
• Ureteropelvic obstruction or stenosis.

Mechanical obstruction of the meatus and urethra occurs only in boys. Severe vesicoureteric reflux eventually results in upper renal tract dilatation without obstruction.

Tumours

There are two ways in which tumours can cause obstruction:
1. Internal: tumours within the urinary tract wall or lumen (e.g. bladder carcinoma). These occupy the urinary tract lumen, causing direct obstruction.
2. External: pressure from rectal or prostate tumours or from gynaecological malignancies narrows the urinary tract lumen, causing indirect obstruction.

Calculi

Stones in the urinary tract can cause urinary obstruction.

Pregnancy

The high levels of progesterone in pregnancy relax smooth muscle fibres in the renal pelvis and ureters and cause a dysfunctional obstruction. There might also be external compression from the pressure of the enlarging fetus on the ureters.

Hyperplastic lesions

The most common hyperplastic lesion causing urinary obstruction is benign prostatic hypertrophy (BPH).

Inflammation

Any inflammation in the lower urinary tract will cause an obstruction (e.g. urethritis, ureteritis, prostatitis, retroperitoneal fibrosis). Obstruction resolves with the treatment of the inflammation.

Neurogenic disorders

These result from:
• Congenital anomalies affecting the spinal cord (e.g. spina bifida).
• External pressure on the cord or lumbar nerve roots (e.g. meningioma, lumbar disc prolapse).
• Trauma to the spinal cord.

Hydronephrosis

This is dilatation of the renal pelvis and calyces due to obstruction at any point in the urinary tract causing increased pressure above the blockage. It can be:
• Unilateral: caused by an upper urinary tract obstruction. This is detected late because renal function is maintained by the other kidney. Thus, the affected kidney can be severely impaired by the time obstruction is detected.
• Bilateral: because of obstruction in the lower urinary tract. Renal failure develops earlier and prompt intervention is required to prevent chronic renal failure.

Progressive atrophy of the kidney develops as the back pressure from the obstruction is transmitted

- Obstruction at the pyeloureteric junction: hydronephrosis.
- Obstruction of the ureter: hydroureter, eventually developing hydronephrosis.
- Obstruction of the bladder neck/urethra: bladder distension with hypertrophy, eventually leading to hydroureter and thus hydronephrosis.

into the distal parts of the nephron. The glomerular filtration rate (GFR) declines and, if the obstruction is bilateral, the patient goes into renal failure. Progressive damage to the renal structures results in flattening of the calyces with gradual thinning of the renal parenchyma, eventually leaving a cystic thin-walled fibrous sac with no functional capacity.

- Sudden and complete obstruction causes a significant fall in GFR, resulting in acute renal failure.
- Partial or chronic obstruction does not affect the GFR, so renal function is impaired gradually.

Presentation of urinary obstruction
This depends upon the site and cause of the obstruction:

- An acute complete obstruction in the ureters (e.g. due to a stone) causes severe renal colic. If bilateral, the patient is at risk of acute renal failure.
- Gradual obstruction (e.g. prostatic hypertrophy) causes bladder distension with hesitancy, terminal dribbling, poor urine flow and a sense of incomplete voiding.
- A unilateral and partial obstruction causing a hydroureter or hydronephrosis might not be apparent for many years because the unaffected kidney maintains adequate renal function.
- A bilateral and partial obstruction presents with nocturia and polyuria caused by tubular cell dysfunction with an inability to concentrate urine. Other chronic manifestations include renal stones, salt wasting, distal renal tubular acidosis and hypertension. If undiagnosed, the patient develops chronic renal failure.
- A bilateral and complete obstruction presents as anuria or oliguria and must be treated for survival. Following removal of the obstruction, there is massive postobstructive diuresis that leaves the patient susceptible to dehydration. Any general malaise or fever might be a sign of superimposed infection.

In all cases, management must include relief of the obstruction either with a urinary catheter, urinary stent or a nephrostomy (to allow renal function to improve), followed by surgical intervention.

Urolithiasis (urinary calculi)
Incidence and risk factors
Urinary calculi affect 1–5% of the population and are more common in men. They are formed by precipitation of urinary components along with a small core of organic material, and form anywhere along the urinary tract, most commonly in the renal pelvis. Calculi vary in size and number. Risk factors for stone formation include:

- Increased solute in the urine as a result of high plasma levels (e.g. calcium and urate) or abnormal tubular function (e.g. calcium and cysteine).
- Absence of inhibiting substances (e.g. citrate and phosphate).
- Acidic urinary pH, which reduces solubility of a substance in the urine.
- Urinary stasis or obstruction.

Occasionally, a calculus can grow to take up the shape of the renal pelvis and branch into calyces (staghorn calculus). Stone formation is initiated by a core of mucoproteins or urates (nucleation); as more components deposit on the core, the stone gradually increases in size (aggregation). Figure 5.14 lists the different types of stone and their frequency.

Presentation
The clinical presentation includes:

- Renal colic due to the increase in peristalsis in the ureters in response to the passage of small stones along the ureter.

Different types of renal stone and their frequency	
Type	**Frequency (%)**
calcium-containing stones:	
• calcium oxalate	60–70
• calcium phosphate	10–15
complex triple stones (magnesium, aluminium, phosphate)	15
uric acid stones	5
cysteine stones	1–2

Fig. 5.14 Different types of renal stone and their frequency.

- A continuous dull ache in the loins due to kidney stones.
- Strangury: the urge to pass something that will not pass (bladder stone).
- Recurrent and untreatable UTIs, haematuria or renal failure.
- Asymptomatic.

Treatment

Management involves adequate analgesia and a high fluid intake. Stones less than 0.5 cm in diameter usually pass spontaneously; larger stones might require surgical intervention. Treatment options include:

- Percutaneous surgery: endoscopic removal of the stone.
- Extracorporeal lithotripsy: shockwaves are used to fragment the calculi into small pieces which will then pass naturally.

Prevention of renal stones includes:

- A high fluid intake to produce a dilute urine.
- Correction of any underlying metabolic abnormality.
- Open surgical removal.
- Combination of the above.

Inflammation of the urinary tract

Ureteritis

This is inflammation of the ureter and can occur in UTI. Persistent or recurrent infection leads to

chronic inflammation, which has two reaction patterns:

1. Ureteritis folliculitis: lymphocytic aggregation under the epithelium causes elevation of the mucosal surface with a fine granular appearance.
2. Ureteritis cystica: multiple small cysts (1–5 mm) develop from fibrosed clumps of epithelial cells on the surface of the ureteric mucosa. They are thin walled with clear fluid, and project into the lumen.

Cystitis

This is inflammation of the urinary bladder and is common in UTI. It can be acute or chronic. The aetiology and predisposing factors were discussed with UTI (see p. 76). The pathogens that cause cystitis are:

- Most common: *Escherichia coli* and *Proteus* species, followed by *Enterobacter*.
- *Candida albicans* in patients on long-term antibiotics.
- *Cryptococcus* species in immunosuppressed patients.
- *Schistosoma* species, particularly in Middle Eastern countries.
- *Mycobacterium tuberculosis*: tuberculous cystitis usually suggests tuberculosis in the upper urinary tract.

Sterile cystitis can be caused by radiation damage, drugs and instrumentation.

The most serious complication of cystitis is pyelonephritis.

Acute cystitis

In acute cystitis the mucosa becomes hyperaemic, often producing an exudate. There are various forms:

- Haemorrhagic cystitis: occurs if the hyperaemia becomes excessive, resulting in bleeding.
- Exudative cystitis: yellow areas of fibrinous exudate develop on the mucosa.
- Suppurative cystitis: large quantities of exudate accumulate.
- Ulcerative cystitis: large areas of ulceration occur in the bladder mucosa.
- Gangrenous cystitis: as a result of ischaemia, which results in areas of black necrotic bladder mucosa.

Chronic cystitis

This results from recurrent or persistent infection of the bladder. Chronic infection leads to fibrous thickening, so the bladder wall is less distensible. This affects the ability of the bladder to store urine and contract during micturition.

Other types of cystitis

Interstitial cystitis

This type of cystitis is often associated with SLE, so is thought to be an autoimmune condition. As with all autoimmune conditions, it has a much higher incidence in women than in men. It can also result from recurrent and persistent infection that leads to fibrosis of all the layers of the bladder wall. There is often localized ulceration of the mucosa.

Malakoplakia vesicae

This is a very rare form of chronic bacterial cystitis, but it is important because it can mimic a tumour. Raised mucosal plaques of inflammation cells develop on the bladder and ureteric mucosa. These plaques are inflammatory, soft, yellow, 3–5 cm in diameter and are prone to ulceration. On histology the plaques are found to contain foamy macrophages with a granular cytoplasm containing Michaelis–Gutmann bodies and chronic inflammatory cells. Malakoplakia is more common in renal transplant patients.

Presentation and treatment

The classic symptoms of all types of cystitis are:
- Urgency and frequency of micturition.
- Dysuria.
- Lower abdominal pain and tenderness.

There might be associated systemic signs of fever, general malaise and rigors.

Treatment of cystitis involves a 3–5-day course of antibiotics with a high fluid intake. Recurrent infection should always be investigated.

Schistosomiasis (bilharzia)

Schistosomiasis is the most common helminth infection worldwide, although it is rare in the UK. It is endemic in the Middle East, Africa, the Far East and in parts of South America. The pathogen is a blood fluke (*Schistosoma haematobium*). Humans are infected via freshwater snails, which contain cerecariae—parasites in the cercarial phase of development. The schistosomes penetrate intact skin to enter the venous system, and thus migrate to the liver and bladder. They settle in the bladder to lay eggs causing chronic irritation of the transitional cells of the bladder. The eggs are excreted into local water supplies and transmitted through freshwater snails (Fig. 5.15).

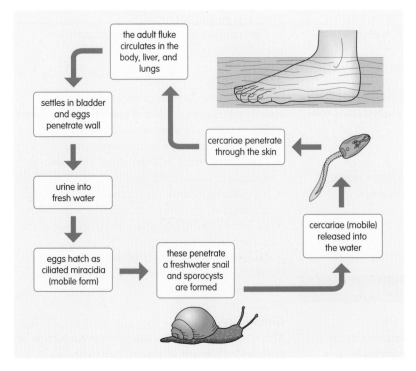

Fig. 5.15 Infestation with *Schistosoma haematobium*.

People infected with cercariae can present with an itchy papular rash accompanied by myalgia, abdominal pain and headache. The most common presentation of infection with *S. haematobium* is recurrent haematuria. Eventually, obstruction within the urinary tract, bladder calcification (predisposing to squamous carcinoma) and renal failure occur.

Diagnosis involves:
- Urine sample to detect the eggs in the urine.
- Enzyme-linked immunosorbent assay (ELISA) to detect a response to infection.

Treatment is with praziquantel given once daily.

Metaplasia associated with bladder extrophy, chronic bladder inflammation and schistosomiasis are premalignant conditions.

Urethral inflammation
The most common pathogens are *E. coli* and *Proteus* species. Ascending infection including cystitis, ureteritis and pyelitis can result.

Acute inflammation of the urethra occurs from infection with a sexually transmitted disease (e.g. *Neisseria gonorrhoeae* or *Chlamydia trachomatis*). (see *Crash course: Endocrine and reproductive system* for further details). Urethritis is seen with conjunctivitis and arthritis in Reiter's disease.

Neoplastic disease of the urinary tract

Tumours of the ureters
These are very rare.

Benign tumours of the ureter
These originate from blood vessels, lymphatics and smooth muscle. A fibroepithelial polyp is a small mass that projects into the lumen. It consists of a clump of vascular connective tissue beneath the ureteric mucosa.

Malignant tumours of the ureters
Primary malignancies are very rare and metastatic disease is relatively more common in the ureters.

Malignant tumours arise from the transitional epithelium lining the ureters and most of the urinary tract. They are usually asymptomatic for many years and are found in 60–70-year-olds. They eventually present as a partial and unilateral obstruction as the ureteric lumen becomes occluded. They often occur in association with multiple tumours of the bladder and renal pelvis (synchronous tumours of the uroepithelium).

Tumours of the bladder
Metaplasia
The transitional cell lining (urothelium) of the bladder can undergo metaplastic changes during any period of infection or inflammation as a result of stones, drugs and radiation. There are three types of metaplasia:

1. Squamous metaplasia: occurs in areas of long-term chronic inflammation in bladder extrophy, bladder calculi, and schistosomiasis. It is a risk factor for squamous cell carcinoma.
2. Intestinal or glandular metaplasia: associated with chronic cystitis and leads to the formation of slit-like glands of columnar epithelium.
3. Nephrogenic metaplasia (rare): associated with chronic infections. The urothelium is transformed to cuboidal epithelium, and must be differentiated from adenocarcinoma.

Benign tumours of the bladder
These are very rare, accounting for 2–3% of bladder epithelial tumours. Transitional cell papilloma can be the first stage (grade I) of transitional cell carcinoma. These papillomas are often multiple and are found all over the mucosal lining. They are small projections (0.5–2.0cm in length) with uniform cellular structure. They attach to the mucosa by a small stalk with a fibrovascular core covered in urothelium.

The other benign lesions are inverted papillomas. These consist of solitary nodules in the mucosa and measure 1–3cm in diameter.

Transitional cell carcinomas
These are malignant tumours that arise from the transitional cell epithelium that lines the bladder. They account for over 90% of bladder epithelial cell tumours, and the number of cases is increasing. They are uncommon under 50 years of age and more commonly affect males (4 males:1 female).

The most common urinary tract malignancy is transitional cell carcinoma and the most common site is the bladder. In countries where schistosomiasis is endemic, squamous cell carcinoma of the bladder is common.

Presentation

The most common presentation of any tumour of the bladder is painless haematuria. This is often accompanied by symptoms of a UTI (i.e. dysuria, frequency and urgency). Symptoms can also be caused by local invasion of the tumour causing ureteric obstruction. Risk factors include:

- Smoking.
- Exposure to chemicals in the rubber industry (e.g. naphthylamine and benzidine).
- Analgesic abuse.

Pathology

There are two main types of transitional cell tumour (Fig. 5.16):

1. Papillary tumour (70%): wart-like lesion covered in a thick layer of urothelium branching off a stalk that attaches it to the mucosa (as described above).
2. Sessile (flat) tumour: plaques of thickened mucosa with a well-defined border.

Both these types of tumour can be in situ or invasive:

- In situ carcinomas: flat lesions that are confined to the mucosa of the upper urinary tract or bladder. They are the precursors of the invasive tumours.
- Invasive tumours: infiltrate the basement membrane of the bladder mucosa and the lamina

propria and can penetrate adjacent structures once through the mucosal wall.

Transitional cell carcinomas can be graded according to the degree of cellular abnormalities on histology:

- Grade I: there is an increase in the number of well-differentiated epithelial cell layers (>7) and there is some cell atypia.
- Grade II: there is an increase in cell layers (>10) and there is a large variation in cell size and in nucleus shape and size (i.e. moderately well differentiated).
- Grade III: the cells have no resemblance to their cells of origin (poorly differentiated), with breakdown of connections between the cells causing them to fragment.

As tumour growth progresses, the relatively benign, well-differentiated papillary growths (grade I) can eventually form solid plaque-like anaplastic tumours (grade III). Grade III tumours are often ulcerated and have penetrated though the bladder muscle wall. They are associated with the worst prognosis.

Carcinomas with over 5% squamous or glandular metaplasia are called mixed tumours.

The TNM system is used for the staging of transitional cell tumours, i.e. to assess the extent of spread (Fig. 5.17). This has been correlated to grade. Tumour spread can be:

- Local: invasion into the bladder wall and to adjacent pelvic structures.
- Distant: lymphatic spread to the periaortic lymph nodes or haematological metastases to the liver and lungs.

Investigation via cystoscopy and biopsy allows histological examination, which confirms whether there is muscle involvement. The distinction between the lamina propria invasion and submucosal invasion is correlated with the prognosis.

Most of the tumours are situated on the posterior and lateral walls of the bladder, and are often multiple. This suggests that the entire epithelium is unstable as a result of the constant exposure to the carcinogens being excreted in urine.

Diagnosis, treatment and prognosis

Diagnosis is made by cytological examination of the urine to check for the presence of malignant cells and by cystoscopy of the lower urinary tract.

Treatment depends upon the stage and histological grade of the tumour:

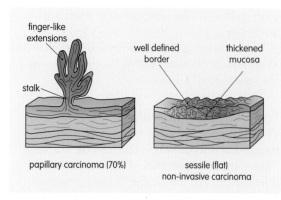

Fig. 5.16 Papillary and sessile transitional cell tumours.

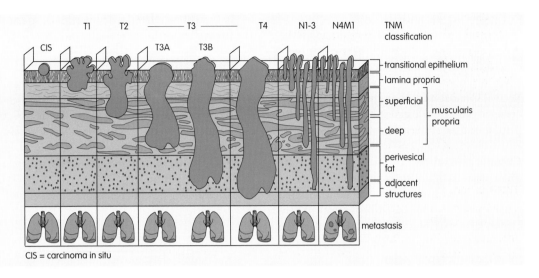

CIS = carcinoma in situ

Fig. 5.17 TNM staging system for transitional cell carcinoma of bladder. T staging decribes tumour invasion of the tissue layers. N staging describes the degree of spread to the lymph nodes: 1 = local nodes; 2 = distant nodes below the diaphragm; 3 = distant nodes on both sides of the diaphragm. M staging describes the presence or absence of metastases: 0 = none; 1 = present (from Bahnson RR 1994 Management of urologic disorders. Mosby Year Book).

- T1 tumours: tumour resection using diathermy (via cystoscopy) with close follow-up.
- T2/3 tumours: radiotherapy and cystectomy.
- T4 tumours: palliative radiotherapy.

The average 5-year survival rate is 80% if the bladder wall is not involved and 5% if there is local invasion on presentation. Patients with fixed tumours and metastases have a median survival of 1 year.

Squamous cell carcinoma

These usually arise in areas of squamous metaplasia of the bladder mucosa and account for <10% of bladder carcinomas. Risk factors include bladder extrophy, chronic inflammation, calculi and schistosomiasis, which cause chronic irritation to the transitional cells of the bladder, leading to squamous metaplasia. This becomes dysplastic, resulting in carcinoma in situ, which can progress to invasive squamous cell carcinoma.

The tumours are solid, ulcerative, invasive and fungating masses, and are often very extensive on discovery. Their prognosis is worse than that of transitional cell carcinoma.

Adenocarcinoma

This is rare in the bladder and usually occurs in the urachal remnants, at the apex of the bladder. Histology shows metaplasia of the transitional epithelium or cystitis cystica.

The most common site for bladder tumours to develop is the posterior and lateral walls (70%) followed by the trigone and bladder neck (20%).

Disorders of the prostate

Prostatitis

There are three subgroups of inflammation of the prostate.

Acute prostatitis

The main pathogens are *E. coli*, *Proteus* and *Staphylococcus* species, and sexually transmitted pathogens including *Chlamydia trachomatis* and gonorrhoea. Inflammation can be focal or diffuse. Infection is usually spread from an acute infection in the urethra or bladder because of:
- Intraprostatic reflux of urine.
- Intraprostatic catheterization.
- Surgical manipulation of the urethra (e.g. cystoscopy).

Occasionally, acute prostatitis is caused by a blood-borne infection.

On histology there is an acute inflammatory infiltrate of neutrophils and damaged cells, often resulting in abscess formation.

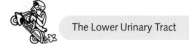

Patients present with:
- General symptoms: malaise, rigors and fever.
- Local symptoms: difficulty in passing urine, dysuria and perineal tenderness.

Rectal examination reveals a soft, tender, and enlarged prostate. Diagnosis is based on the clinical features and a positive urine culture.

Chronic prostatitis

This results from inadequately treated acute infection. This can occur because some antibiotics cannot penetrate the prostate effectively. There is often a history of recurrent prostatic and urinary tract infections. Causative pathogens are the same as for acute prostatic infection.

Patients present with dysuria and low back and perineal pain, with no preceding acute phase. Some patients are asymptomatic.

Chronic prostatitis is difficult to diagnose and treat. Diagnosis is confirmed by:
- Histology showing neutrophils, plasma cells and lymphocytes.
- A positive culture from a sample of prostatic secretion.

Tuberculosis is a cause of chronic infection and can affect the kidneys or epididymis. Histology reveals focal areas of caseation and giant-cell infiltrates.

Chronic non-bacterial prostatitis

This is the most common type of prostatitis and results in enlargement of the prostate, which can obstruct the urethra. The usual pathogen is *Chlamydia trachomatis* so, typically, sexually active men are affected. Often there is no history of recurrent UTIs.

Presentation is similar to that of chronic prostatitis and histology shows fibrosis as a result of chronic inflammation.

Diagnosis is confirmed by the presence of 15 white blood cells per high power field (this indicates inflammation) and repeated negative bacterial cultures (excludes infection).

Benign prostatic hypertrophy (BPH)
Incidence

BPH is detectable to some extent in nearly all men over the age of 60. It is a non-neoplastic enlargement of the prostate gland, which can eventually lead to bladder outflow obstruction. The cause is unknown, but might be related to levels of male sex hormones (testosterone).

Presentation

Symptoms develop as the enlarging gland compresses the prostatic urethra and the periurethral glands (known as the median lobe) swell, affecting the bladder sphincter mechanism. Patients present with 'prostatism', a triad of:
- Difficulty or hesitancy in starting to urinate.
- A poor stream.
- Dribbling postmicturition, frequency and nocturia.

Examination must include:
- Abdominal examination for an enlarged palpable bladder.
- Digital rectal examination for the prostate, which is firm, smooth and rubbery.

Untreated BPH can present with acute urinary retention, which is accompanied by a distended and tender bladder and a desparate urge to pass urine. Alternatively, the patient might have progressive bladder distension, leading to chronic painless retention and overflow incontinence. If undetected, BPH can lead to bilateral upper tract obstruction and renal impairment, with the patient presenting in chronic renal failure (see Chapter 6).

Pathology

There is hyperplasia of both the lateral lobes and the median lobes (these lie behind the urethra), leading to compression of the urethra and therefore bladder outflow obstruction. Within the prostate there are solid nodules of fibromuscular material and cystic regions. Histology shows hyperplasia of the:
- Stroma (smooth muscle and fibrous tissue).
- Glands, often with areas of infarction and necrosis.

Complications

The complications of BPH develop from prolonged obstruction to urine flow. There is compensatory hypertrophy of the bladder as a result of the high pressures that develop within the bladder (Fig. 5.18).

Treatment
- Medical treatment: symptoms can be improved with α-blockers (which relax smooth muscle at

Fig. 5.18 Complications of benign prostatic hypertrophy. (A) Bands of thickened smooth muscle fibre cause trabeculation of the bladder wall. (B) Diverticula can develop on the external surface of the bladder. (C) Dilatation of the bladder once the muscle becomes hypotonic. (D) Formation of hydroureters resulting in the reflux of urine up to the renal pelvis. (E) Bilateral hydronephrosis. (F) Kidney infection, stones, calculi and renal failure.

the bladder neck, thus improving urinary flow rate) and antiandrogens such as finasteride. Finasteride is a 5α-reductase inhibitor that prevents the conversion of testosterone to the more potent androgen dihydrotestosterone. Dihydrotestosterone promotes growth and enlargement of the prostate; inhibition of its production causes gradual reduction in prostate volume, thereby improving urinary flow rate and obstructive symptoms.

- Surgical treatment: transurethral resection of the prostate (TURP) is quick and safe with a low mortality and a good success rate.

Carcinoma of the prostate
Incidence and risk factors
Prostate cancer is the third most common cancer in men (after cancer of the lung and stomach), accounting for 8% of all cancers in men. It is a disease of elderly men, occurring in one in ten men of 70 years of age. It is rare under 55 years of age and has a strong hereditary component.

The cause is unknown, but there is a link between androgenic hormones and tumour growth. The lesions are most commonly found in the periphery of the posterior part of the prostate compared with the more central and lateral location of BPH—these areas have different embryological origins and often both conditions coexist.

Presentation
Patients present with symptoms of UTI, prostatism or metastatic disease in the bone (usually the spine) causing bone pain. Carcinoma can be found coincidentally in autopsies of elderly men who were asymptomatic. About 25% of patients have symptoms of metastatic disease on presentation (anaemia, ureteric obstruction or bone pain that is worse at night).

Pathology
The tumours range from well-differentiated single nodules to anaplastic and diffuse involvement of all lobes of the gland. The Gleeson classification is used to grade the tumours on histological appearance. Grade 1 is a well-differentiated tumour composed of uniform tumour cells whereas grade 5 is an anaplastic diffuse tumour with cells showing great variation in their structure and a high mitotic rate.

As for transitional cell carcinoma of the bladder, stage is determined by the universal TNM system:
- T_1: unsuspected impalpable tumour.
- T_2: the tumour is confined to the prostate.
- T_3: there is local extension of the tumour beyond the prostatic capsule.
- T_4: the tumour has fixed to other local structures.

Tumour spread can be by:
- Local invasion of adjacent structures, including the bladder and ureters.
- Lymphatic spread to the iliac and periaortic nodes.

- Haematogenous spread to the bones of the spine and pelvis and occasionally to the lungs and liver.

Diagnosis

- Digital rectal examination: hard and irregular prostate.
- Ultrasound: used to define a prostatic mass.
- Prostatic specific antigen (PSA) level in the blood: this increases in prostate cancer, but a normal result does not exclude the presence of cancer.
- Serum prostatic acid phosphatase: this also increases, especially if there are metastases.
- Radiographs and bone scans: used to stage the tumour. Osteosclerotic lesions on radiographs and increased isotope uptake on bone scans are seen if there is metastatic spread (see Chapter 8).

Treatment and prognosis

Treatment options include surgery, hormone therapy and radiotherapy. Before treatment is started, a histological diagnosis of prostatic carcinoma is required. The specimen is taken by transurethral or transrectal biopsy. Treatment depends upon the stage of the tumour:

- T1/T2 staged tumours: surgical resection of the prostate (prostatectomy). TURP might also be required in advanced metastatic disease to relieve the symptoms of urethral obstruction.
- Local radiotherapy can be used if the patient is unfit for surgery, and to treat local or distant spread of the tumour. It can provide useful palliation for bony metastases.
- Advanced tumours: hormonal treatments are important. Testosterone promotes tumour growth. Thus, removal of both testes (orchidectomy) blocks the source of testosterone, causing the tumour to shrink. This is rarely used. Luteinizing-hormone-releasing hormone (LHRH) analogues (e.g. buserelin) prevent testosterone release. They are equally effective and are increasingly used. Antiandrogens such as cyproterone acetate are also used to block testosterone action.

Prognosis depends on stage. The 5-year survival rate for T1 tumours is 75–90%. However, the 5-year survival falls to 30–45% if there is local or metastastic spread.

- Explain what the 'trigone' is and how it differs from the rest of the bladder.
- Name three differences between the external and internal urethral sphincters.
- Outline the function of the detrusor and sphincter muscles, and their innervation.
- Summarize the common causes and points of neurological damage within the micturition path.
- Describe 'spinal shock'.
- Outline the difference between a hydroureter and a megaloureter.
- Explain how diverticulae develop, where they occur and their long-term effects.
- Name three causes of urinary tract obstruction. List the imaging techniques you would use to investigate obstruction.
- Describe how clinical presentation of urinary obstruction is influenced by the site and cause of the obstruction.
- Discuss how bilateral hydronephrosis differs in presentation from unilateral hydronephrosis.
- Summarize the factors influencing stone formation. What is the management for urinary stones?
- Outline the mechanism by which schistosomiasis increases the risk of bladder cancer.
- Compare and contrast the three types of inflammation affecting the prostate.
- Define BPH, explaining the histological changes.
- Explain how treatment and prognosis differ according to the stage of prostate cancer.

CLINICAL ASSESSMENT

Introduction

There are numerous presenting complaints in renal disease. In this chapter each will be dealt with individually. Many of these, however, are non-specific and renal disease can be asymptomatic until a very late stage. It is therefore essential to have a routine screening procedure of:

- Blood pressure measurement.
- Urinalysis (midstream urine).

Blood and urine abnormalities

Haematuria

Blood in the urine can be:

- Microscopic: blood is visible only under a microscope or on dipstick analysis.
- Macroscopic ('frank' haematuria): blood is visible with the naked eye (>5 red blood cells per high-power field).

The degree of haematuria does not always reflect the severity of the underlying disorder.

Causes

Causes of haematuria are:

- Renal causes: glomerular disease such as primary glomerulonephritis (e.g. IgA nephropathy), disorders secondary to systemic illness (e.g. vasculitis, systemic lupus erythematosus—SLE), carcinoma (both renal and transitional cell), trauma, cystic disease, emboli.
- Extrarenal causes: urinary tract infection (UTI)*, ureteral calculi*, prostatic hypertrophy*, carcinoma of the bladder*, renal stone*, trauma, urethritis, catheterization, post-cyclophosphamide.
- Systemic causes: coagulation disorders, sickle-cell trait or disease.
- Others: anticoagulant drugs.

(*indicates the most common causes)

Dipsticks detect haemoglobin (not red blood cells) and will give positive results if there is intravascular haemolysis (i.e. red blood cell breakdown in the blood). This is because haemoglobin is filtered freely by glomeruli (haemoglobinuria). This can occur physiologically, after heavy exercise, during pregnancy or with prosthetic heart valves. If haemolysis is severe (i.e. in haemolytic crisis), the urine can become red.

Other conditions can cause a red–brown discoloration of the urine that can be confused with haematuria (e.g. porphyria, myoglobinuria, ingestion of some foods (beetroot) or drugs (phenolphthalein)).

Diagnostic approach

Figure 6.1 shows the common sites of lesions causing haematuria and the investigative approach for haematuria is shown in Fig. 6.2. A flow chart summarizing further investigation of haematuria if the IVP or ultrasound result is abnormal is given in Fig. 6.3. The significance of urinalysis is summarized in Fig. 6.4.

Proteinuria

Proteinuria is the presence of excess protein in the urine. It is usually assessed using a dipstick, which detects protein levels above 300mg/L. 'Microalbuminuria' is the presence of excess urinary protein (usually albumin) but in amounts insufficient to cause a positive dipstick analysis. Proteinuria is measured as the protein concentration on a 'spot' urine sample or the amount excreted in 24h (the amount of protein excreted varies through the day). Urine usually contains <20mg/L of albumin and <200mg/day of protein (exact values vary from laboratory to laboratory according to methods used to measure protein). The presence of protein is associated with nephropathy in diabetes and increased cardiovascular risk in hypertension and ischaemic heart disease.

Causes

Causes of proteinuria are summarized, together with relevant investigations, in Fig. 6.5.

Nephrotic syndrome

This is characterized by >3g/day proteinuria, which causes a decrease in serum albumin

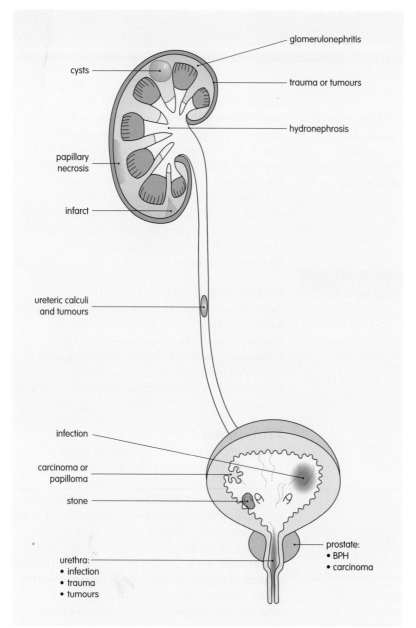

Fig. 6.1 Common sites of lesions causing haematuria. BPH, benign prostatic hypertrophy.

glomerulonephritis

cysts

trauma or tumours

hydronephrosis

papillary necrosis

infarct

ureteric calculi and tumours

infection

carcinoma or papilloma

stone

prostate:
• BPH
• carcinoma

urethra:
• infection
• trauma
• tumours

(hypoalbuminaemia) and hence oedema. It is associated with an increase in cholesterol (hypercholesterolaemia). Primary nephrotic syndrome results from diseases arising in the glomerulus. These include:
- Commonly, minimal change glomerulonephritis, membranous glomerulonephritis, membranoproliferative glomerulonephritis, focal segmental glomerulosclerosis.
- Rarely, other types of glomerulonephritis.

Causes of secondary nephrotic syndrome are diabetic nephropathy, drugs (captopril, NSAIDs), amyloidosis, sickle-cell disease, malaria and vasculitis (SLE).

Diagnostic approach
After initial assessment using urine dipstick, specialist investigations are performed to exclude systemic diseases, drugs and toxins as the cause of proteinuria. This is summarized in Fig. 6.5.

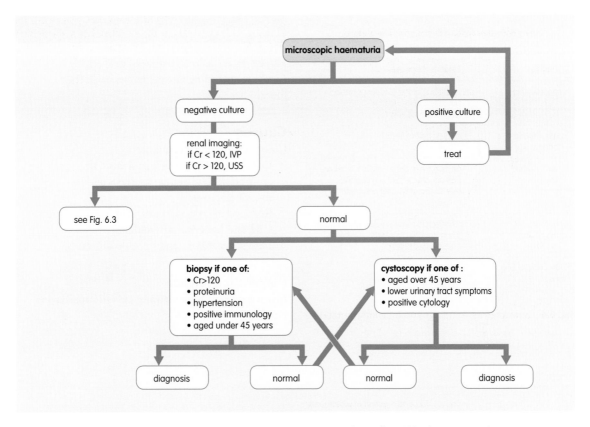

Fig. 6.2 Investigation of haematuria. Cr, creatinine; IVP, intravenous pyelography; USS, ultrasonography.

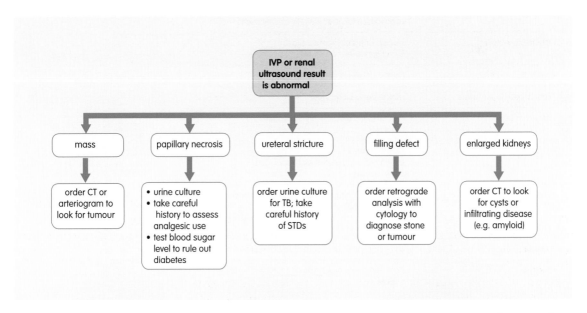

Fig. 6.3 Further investigation of haematuria when the IVP or ultrasound result is abnormal. CT, computed tomography; IVP, intravenous pyelography; STDs, sexually transmitted diseases; TB, tuberculosis (from Green HL 1996 Clinical medicine, 2nd edn. Mosby Year Book).

Urine analysis—possible findings and interpretation

Findings	Possible diagnoses
clots in urine	carcinoma of the bladder or kidney; clot colic is also a feature of IgA nephropathy
albuminuria and haematuria	intrinsic renal disease
red blood cell casts	glomerulonephritis—red cell casts are pathognomic of active glomerular bleeding (e.g. IgA, nephropathy, vasculitis)
haematuria, pyuria and white blood cell casts	renal tubulointerstitial disease; this is a non-specific diagnosis (i.e. pyelonephritis)
dysmorphic red cells	glomerular bleeding (i.e. glomerulonephritis)

Fig. 6.4 Urine analysis—findings and their interpretations.

Hyperuricaemia

Hyperuricaemia is an excess of uric acid (end-product of purine degradation) in the blood.

Causes
Causes of hyperuricaemia are:
- Overproduction of uric acid: seen in lymphoma, leukaemia, psoriasis and muscle necrosis.
- Reduced excretion of uric acid: seen in gout, CRF and hyperparathyroidism.
- Drugs: cytotoxins and thiazide diuretics.

Diagnostic approach
Investigation of hyperuricaemia is summarized in Fig. 6.6.

Causes and investigation of proteinuria

Cause	Investigation
urinary tract infection	midstream urine sample and culture
diabetic nephropathy	blood glucose levels (glucose tolerance test); examination for other diabetic complications
glomerulonephritis	biopsy (for histological diagnosis); blood pressure
nephrotic syndrome	cholesterol levels, oedema
congestive cardiac failure	clinical signs, blood pressure
hypertension	regular blood pressure measurements; renal biopsy
myeloma	full blood count; serum and urine protein electrophoresis; bone marrow biopsy
amyloid	biopsy and Congo red staining; look for associated splenomegaly
pregnancy	HCG pregnancy test
pyrexia	core temperature measurement at regular intervals
exercise	urine sample on waking; to be repeated following exercise
postural proteinuria (rare if >30 years old)	urine sample on waking; repeated at mid-day
vaginal mucus contaminant	repeat urine sample, with sterile technique

Fig. 6.5 Causes and investigation of proteinuria. hCG, human chorionic gonadotrophin.

Fig. 6.6 Investigation of hyperuricaemia. *Both a xanthine oxidase inhibitor and a uricosuric agent are needed in tophaceous gout. Xanthine oxidase is an enzyme in the metabolic pathway that produces urate from purines (from Green HL 1996 Clinical medicine, 2nd edn. Mosby Year Book).

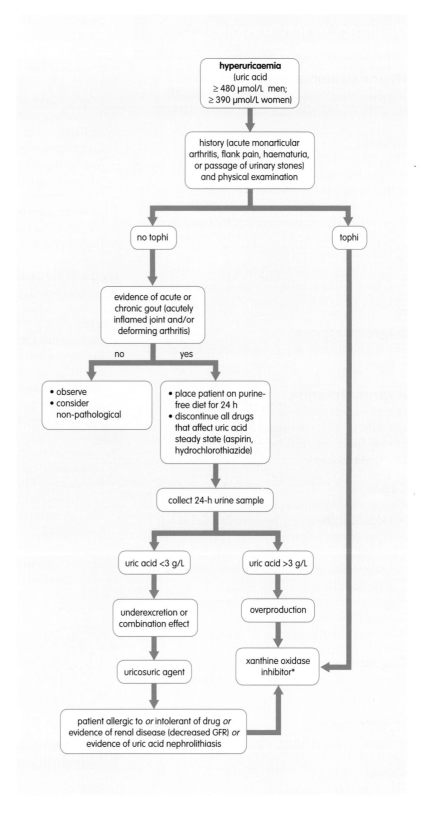

Disorders of serum sodium and potassium

Hyponatraemia

In hyponatraemia plasma $[Na^+]$ is <130mmol/L and there is a decreased solute:water ratio in the ECF.

Causes

The causes of hyponatraemia are:
- Diuretics (mainly thiazides).
- Water overload or retention.
- Increased antidiuretic hormone (ADH) secretion.
- Increased plasma osmolarity (e.g. caused by mannitol, glucose).
- Increased protein or lipids (pseudohyponatraemia). Here, there is less sodium relative to the increase in protein or lipids, giving the impression of a low sodium.

Diagnostic approach

The diagnostic approach to hyponatraemia is shown in Fig. 6.7.

Hypernatraemia

In hypernatraemia the serum sodium is >140mmol/L and there is an increase in solute to water ratio in body fluids and increased serum osmolality (>300mOsmol/kg).

Causes

The causes of hypernatraemia are:
- Osmotic diuresis (e.g. uncontrolled diabetes).
- Fluid loss without replacement (sweating, burns, vomiting).
- Diabetes insipidus (suspect if lots of dilute urine is produced).
- Incorrect intravenous fluid replacement (i.e. hypertonic fluids).
- Primary aldosteronism.

Diagnostic approach

The diagnostic approach to hypernatraemia is shown in Fig. 6.8.

Hypokalaemia

In hypokalaemia plasma $[K^+]$ is <3.5mmol/L.

Causes

Hypokalaemia is caused by:
- Renal losses due to diuretics, excess mineralocorticoids (Conn's syndrome), magnesium deficiency, renal tubular defects (e.g. renal tubular acidosis), reduced intake or metabolic alkalosis (e.g. vomiting).
- Extrarenal losses due to diarrhoea, laxative abuse, vomiting (pyloric stenosis), profuse sweating, colonic villous adenoma or biliary drainage.
- Transcellular shift due to insulin, metabolic alkalosis, catecholamines and other sympathomimetics, rapid proliferation of cells (e.g. treatment of pernicious anaemia with vitamin B_{12}), or periodic paralysis.

Diagnostic approach

An algorithm for the investigation of hypokalaemia is shown in Fig. 6.9.

Hyperkalaemia

In hyperkalaemia, plasma $[K^+]$ >5.5mmol/L.

Causes

Hyperkalaemia can result from:
- Reduced renal excretion: due to renal failure, mineralocorticoid deficiency (e.g. Addison's disease), potassium-sparing diuretics or renal tubular defects.
- Increased plasma load due to dietary changes or cellular tissue breakdown.
- Transcellular shift due to metabolic acidosis, insulin deficiency, exercise or drugs (e.g. digoxin).
- Pseudohyperkalaemia due to efflux from cells (e.g. trauma during venepuncture, prolonged storage, haemolysis), thrombolysis or leucocytosis.

Diagnostic approach

An algorithm for the investigation of hyperkalaemia is shown in Fig. 6.10.

 As K^+ is predominantly intracellular, plasma $[K^+]$ is a poor predictor of total body K^+.

Renal failure

Uraemia

Uraemia is the accumulation of nitrogenous metabolic waste products in the blood (i.e. urea and

Fig. 6.7 Diagnostic approach to hyponatraemia. ECF, extracellular fluid; SIADH, syndrome of inappropriate ADH secretion; TURP, transurethral resection of the prostate.

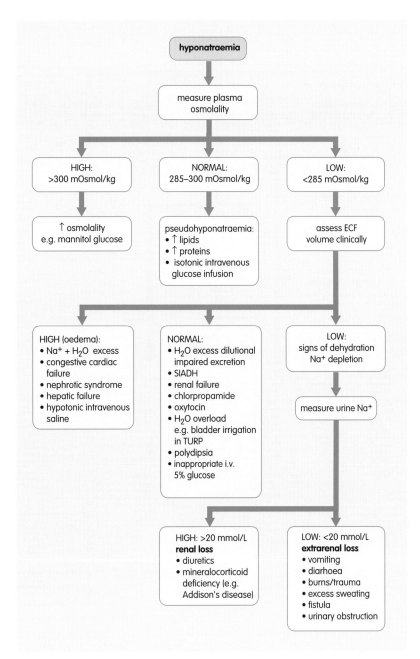

creatinine). The kidneys are unable to filter and excrete these products.

- Acute renal failure: uraemia developing rapidly within a few days.
- Chronic renal failure: uraemia of gradual onset—over a period of months to years.

Acute renal failure (ARF)

Causes of acute renal failure can be classified as prerenal, renal and postrenal.

Prerenal causes of ARF are:
- Hypovolaemia (e.g. shock, burns, dehydration, sepsis, haemorrhage), resulting in decreased effective circulating volume.
- Reduced effective circulating volume (e.g. in congestive cardiac failure, liver disease).
- Drugs altering renal haemodynamics (e.g. non-steroidal anti-inflammatory drugs—NSAIDs, angiotensin-converting

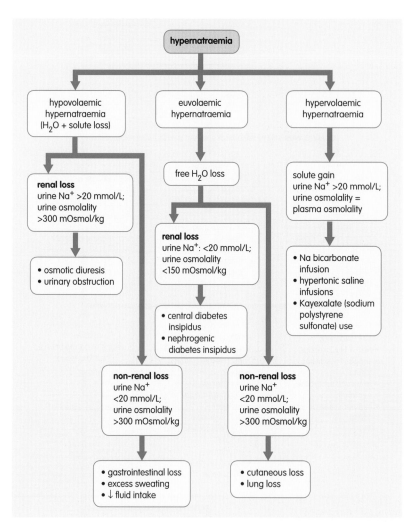

Fig. 6.8 Diagnostic approach to hypernatraemia.

enzyme inhibitors, antihypertensives, ciclosporin).
- Renal artery stenosis or emboli.

Renal causes of ARF are:
- Acute tubular necrosis: any untreated prerenal cause, drug toxicity (e.g. gentamicin, acyclovir, methotrexate) and toxins (e.g. myoglobinuria and lipopolysaccharide in Gram-negative sepsis).
- Acute glomerulonephritis.
- Acute interstitial nephritis (due to drugs, infections, hypercalcaemia, multiple myeloma).
- Vasculitis.
- Hypertension.
- Emboli (such as thrombi, cholesterol).
- Acute cortical necrosis (severe shock left untreated).

Postrenal or obstructive causes of ARF are:
- Bladder outflow obstruction (benign prostatic hypertrophy or urethral strictures).
- Retroperitoneal fibrosis.
- Tumour (prostate, bladder, or extrinsic compression by gynaecological malignancy).
- Stone (would need to be bilateral to cause ARF).

Note: Obstruction must occur in both kidneys or in a single functioning kidney for renal failure to occur.

Diagnostic approach
Basic investigation of renal failure includes urine tests (dipstick, microscopy, culture, cytology), blood tests and radiology (of the kidney, ureter and bladder—KUB—and IVU). In ARF, the following biochemical changes occur:

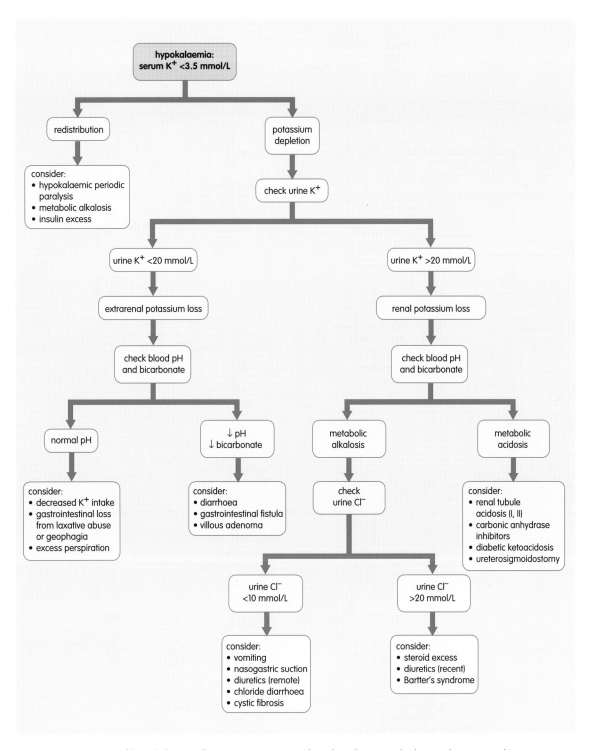

Fig. 6.9 Investigation of hypokalaemia (from Green HL 1996 Clinical medicine, 2nd edn. Mosby Year Book).

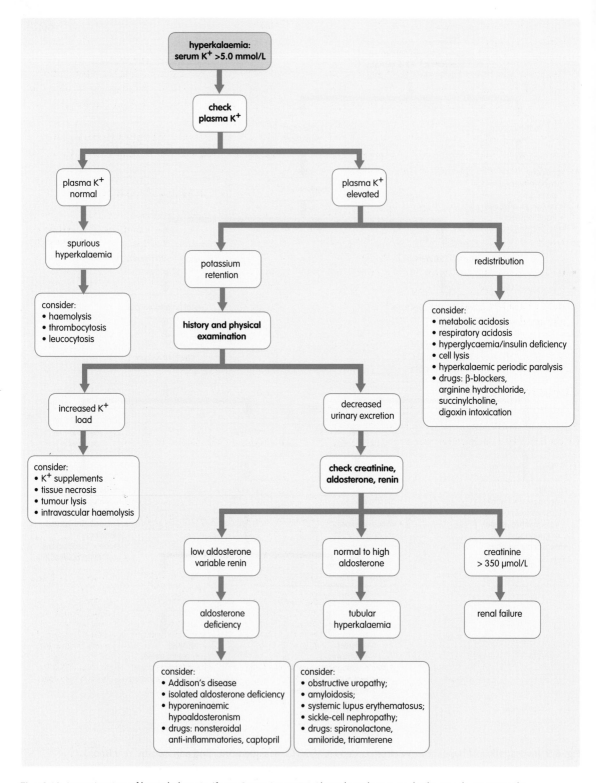

Fig. 6.10 Investigation of hyperkalaemia (from Green HL 1996 Clinical medicine, 2nd edn. Mosby Year Book).

- Increased plasma urea and creatinine concentrations.
- Increased plasma urate.
- Increased plasma concentrations of potassium.
- Metabolic acidosis and an increased anion gap.
- Increased plasma phosphate and decreased plasma calcium (less marked than in CRF).
- Decreased plasma sodium can occur.
- Changes in urine biochemistry: these depend on whether prerenal or renal failure exists (Fig. 6.11).

In addition, some serological tests can help clarify the diagnosis:
- Antinuclear antibodies (ANA): systemic lupus erythematosus (SLE)-associated nephritis.
- Cryoglobulin titre: cryoglobulinaemia.
- Complement levels: SLE-associated nephritis, membranoproliferative and acute glomerulonephritis.

Figure 6.12 gives clues to help in the diagnosis of ARF and its possible causes.

Chronic renal failure

Chronic renal failure (CRF) is irreversible impaired renal function. It can result from renal disease or be secondary to other systemic diseases.

Causes

Causes of CRF are:
- **Renal:** glomerulonephritis, chronic pyelonephritis, bladder or urethral obstruction, polycystic kidneys, interstitial nephritis, amyloid, myeloma, renal vascular disease, Alport's syndrome.
- **Extrarenal:** diabetes mellitus, hypertension (expecially if accelerated—malignant), heart

Urine biochemistry results		
Test	Prerenal failure	Renal failure (acute tubular) necrosis)
urine osmolality (mOsm/kg H_2O)	>500	<350
urine sodium (mmol/L)	<20	>40
urine/serum creatinine	>40	<20
urine/serum osmolality	>1.5	<1.2
fractional excreted sodium	<1	>1
renal failure index	↑urea >creatinine	↑urea ↑creatinine

Fig. 6.11 Urine biochemistry results.

Clues to help in diagnosis of acute renal failure and its possible causes			
	Prerenal failure	Renal failure	Postrenal failure
History	thirst; weight loss; potential for volume loss (e.g. surgery, diuretics) ineffective circulating volume	previous abnormal urinalysis; exposure to toxic agents; hypertension; new medications	frequency; hesitancy; nocturia; history of nephrolithiasis or neoplasms; renal colic especially if only one kidney
Physical examination	signs of dehydration; hypotension; hypovolaemia; ↓BP = postural drop; ↑pulse; ↓jugular venous pulse	hypertension; physical signs (e.g. skin lesions of vasculitis)	distended bladder; enlarged prostate
Urinalysis	↑urine osmolality and high specific gravity; ↓urine Na⁺ and fractional excreted Na⁺; ↑urine:serum creatinine	proteinuria; haematuria; pyuria; renal tubular epithelial cells in urinary sediment; casts and their nature	crystalluria (suggests renal calculus)

Fig. 6.12 Clues to help in diagnosis of acute renal failure and its possible causes.

failure, SLE, gout, hypercalcaemia, renovascular disease (atheroma), vasculitis.
- **Drugs:** gold, penicillamine, ciclosporin A, analgesics.

Diagnostic approach

The diagnostic approach to CRF can involve:
- **Urine:** urinalysis (haematuria, glycosuria, proteinuria), microscopy (white cells, eosinophilia, granular casts, red cell casts, red cells), biochemistry (24-h creatinine clearance, 24-h protein excretion, urinary electrolytes, osmolality, protein electrophoresis).
- **Blood:** urea and creatinine, electrolytes, glucose, calcium (decreased), phosphate (increased), urate (increased), protein, osmolality, full blood count, erythrocyte sedimentation rate (ESR), protein electrophoresis, autoantibody screen, complement components, test for sickle-cell disease.
- **Radiology:** ultrasound (to assess kidney size), CT, plain radiography of the abdomen. Hand radiographs can show evidence of osteodystrophy.
- **Renal biopsy:** consider if kidneys are of normal size and the cause of CRF is not clear from other investigations.

When approaching a patient with renal failure, always ask:
- What is the patient's blood volume?
- Is there an obstruction? (this alters renal perfusion).
- Does the patient have an infection?
- What is the kidney size? (if they are small, consider a diagnosis of CRF).

Renal calculi

Overview

Kidney stone disease arises from the formation and movement of stones within the urinary tract. It is more common in males. Different types of stones can form:
- Calcium-containing stones are the most common. They are made of calcium oxalate (spiky), hydroxyapatite, phosphate (smooth and large).

- Uric acid stones (smooth, brown and soft).
- Struvite or infection stones.
- Cysteine stones (yellow and crystalline).

There is no relation between the size of the stones and the severity of the symptoms.

Causes

Causes of kidney stones are:
- Hypercalciuria (of which hypercalcaemia is the sole cause).
- Hyperuricosuria (of which hyperuricaemia is the main cause).
- Hyperoxaluria.
- Cystinuria.
- Infection.
- Renal tubular acidosis.
- Renal disease (e.g. polycystic kidneys).
- Dehydration: a concentrated urine is produced, which increases the risk of stone formation.

Diagnostic approach
History

Ask about the following:
- Diet: high dietary calcium intake (e.g. milk, cheese), high salt instake (calcium is excreted in parallel with sodium in the kidney), high dietary oxalate intake (e.g. spinach, rhubarb, tea).
- Fluid intake and urine volume.
- Chronic diarrhoea: Crohn's disease or dehydration.
- Personal or family history of gout.
- Family history of renal calculi.
- Number of previous urinary tract infections.
- Medications: check for antacid therapy (contains large amounts of absorbable calcium) and long-term antibiotic therapy.
- Past urological history.

Symptoms

In acute presentation, pain is usually colicky and localized to one quadrant of the abdomen, radiating from loin to groin. The patient appears sweaty, pale and restless, with nausea and vomiting.

Examination and investigation

Examinations and investigations for renal calculi should include:
- Looking for clinical evidence of gout.
- Excluding hypercalcaemia and investigating cause if found (e.g. primary hyperparathyroidism).

- Urinalysis: identify and quantify the amount of calcium, oxalate, urate or cysteine in the urine. Is there any haematuria?
- Stone analysis: ask patient to retain voided stones for biochemical testing or X-ray crystallography.
- Imaging: radiographs showing the kidneys, ureters and bladder (KUB), intravenous urography (IVU) and abdominal ultrasound (less helpful, but might show dilatation of obstructed kidney or acoustic shadow from a stone).

Figure 6.13 shows an algorithm for urinary investigations of a patient with calcium kidney stones.

Treatment

Acute episodes are treated with analgesia and increased fluid intake. Urine should be 'sieved' to collect any stones passed for analysis (most pass spontaneously). If obstruction or infection develops, the stones must be removed urgently. In the long term, the mainstay of treatment is a high fluid intake; thiazides can be used in hypercalcuria as they decrease urinary calcium excretion. Allopurinol is used for hyperuricaemia, and penicillamine for cysteinuria.

- Kidney stones cause loin pain.
- Ureteric stones cause renal colic.
- Bladder stones cause 'strangulation', i.e. the desire to pass the stone, but being unable to do so by voiding.

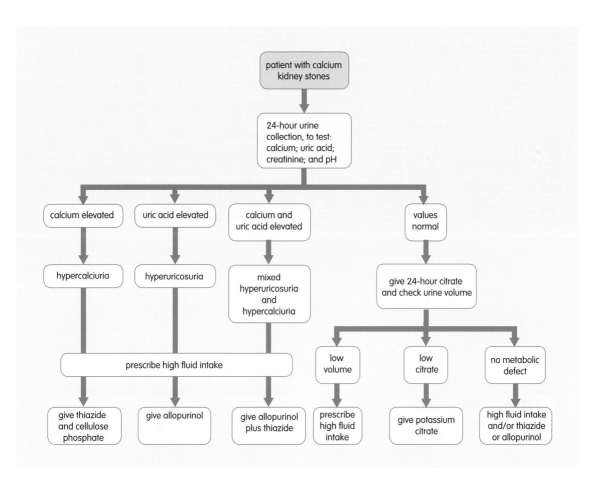

Fig. 6.13 Urinary investigations of a patient with calcium kidney stones (from Green HL 1996 Clinical medicine, 2nd edn. Mosby Year Book).

Urinary incontinence

Urinary incontinence is the involuntary loss of urine. It affects more women than men and is a socially distressing condition. There are several different types.

Stress incontinence ('sphincter insufficiency')

This is involuntary loss of urine associated with an increase in intra-abdominal pressure (e.g. cough). It is caused by:

- Pelvic floor laxity (usually seen in multiparous women).
- Bladder neck sphincter impairment (more common in middle-aged, obese, multiparous women).
- Surgery affecting the urethra or prostate causing damage or weakness to the external sphincter.

Urge incontinence ('detrusor instability')

This is involuntary loss of urine, with the urge to void. There is an urgent 'need to go'. It is due to sensory or motor dysfunction of the bladder. Causes include:

- Inflammation or infection of the lower urinary tract.
- Bladder hyperreflexia.
- Stroke.
- Parkinson's disease.
- Alzheimer's disease.
- Brain tumour.
- Old age.
- Herniated spinal disc.
- Detrusor overactivity caused by a foreign body, stone or urethritis.
- Benign prostatic hypertrophy and obstruction (can cause bladder hypersensitivity).
- Loop diuretics.
- Cough or sneeze.

 The detrusor muscle is the bladder muscle and contracts to cause voiding. This is an automatic reflex, triggered by filling of the bladder to a critical pressure.

Overflow incontinence

This is involuntary leakage of urine when the bladder is full. It is usually due to chronic urine retention secondary to obstruction or an atonic bladder. The causes are:

- Outlet obstruction: faecal impaction, benign prostatic hypertrophy (enlarged prostate).
- Underactive detrusor muscle.
- Bladder neck stricture.
- Urethral stricture.
- α-adrenergic agonists.
- Intra- or postoperative overdistension.
- Use of anticholinergics, calcium channel blockers, sedatives.
- Bladder denervation following surgery.

Total incontinence

This is continuous loss of urine with no voluntary control. The causes are:

- Congenital.
- Secondary to paraplegia, multiple sclerosis, spina bifida.
- Trauma to the external sphincter, bladder neck and perineal muscles.
- Fistula secondary to radiation, surgery, tumour, invasive neoplasms, obstetric injury.

Reflex incontinence

This is involuntary intermittent loss of urine.

Functional incontinence

This is incontinence due to severe cognitive impairment or mobility limitations, preventing use of the toilet. For example, there might be difficulty in reaching the toilet or difficulty in undressing, and the patient is 'caught short'. Bladder function is normal.

Mixed incontinence

In mixed incontinence there is more than one type of problem resulting in incontinence. This is usually seen in elderly patients.

Nocturnal enuresis—bedwetting

Nocturnal enuresis is a childhood disorder. It can be primary (since birth) or secondary (acquired). Both can be due to:

- Uninhibited bladder activity.
- Urinary infection.
- Neurological disease.
- Obstruction.

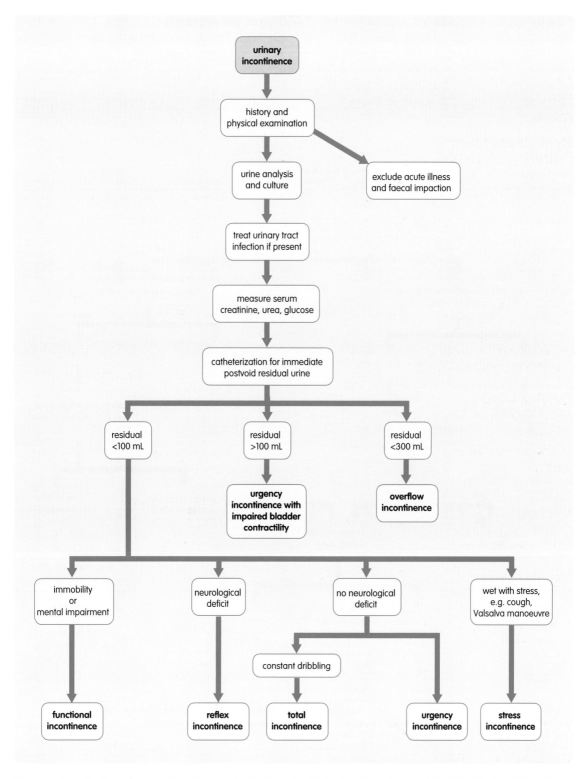

Fig. 6.14 Investigation of urinary incontinence. UTI, urinary tract infection (from Green HL 1996 Clinical medicine, 2nd edn. Mosby Year Book).

After urinary tract infection has been excluded, no further investigation should be performed if the child is less than 5 years old—unless there are any urinary symptoms. Treatment should focus on behaviour therapy, with drug treatment used only as a last resort—sublingual desmopressin is one example.

Diagnostic approach

Figure 6.14 shows an algorithm for the investigation of urinary incontinence.

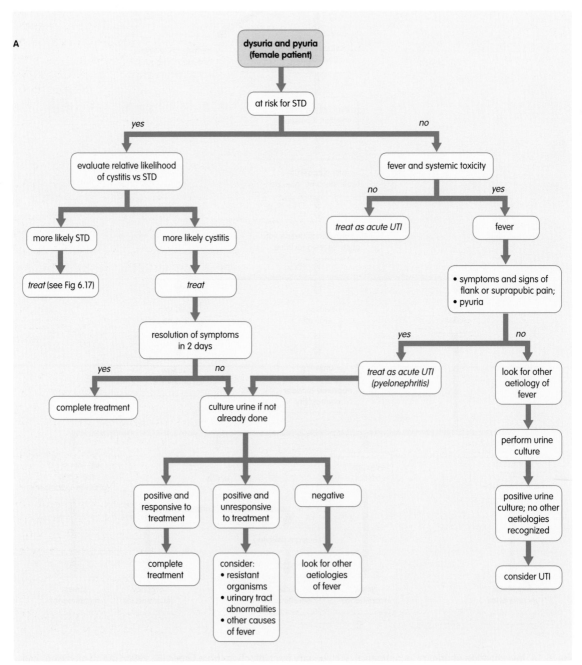

Fig. 6.15 (A) Investigation of urinary tract infection. Dysuria and pyuria in a female patient. STD, sexually transmitted disease; UTI, urinary tract infection (from Green HL 1996 Clinical medicine, 2nd edn. Mosby Year Book).

Urinary tract infection

Overview

Urinary tract infection (UTI) (i.e. $>10^5$ organisms/mL) occurs with or without leucocytes. It is more common in adult females because bacteria can readily access the urinary tract through the short female urethra. UTI results from migration of bacteria through the urethra into the bladder, ureter and kidney. UTIs are also seen in male infants with congenital obstruction and in elderly men with acquired prostatic obstruction.

Different sites of the urinary tract can be affected as follows:

- Upper urinary tract: kidney, resulting in pyelonephritis.
- Lower urinary tract: bladder, resulting in cystitis; prostate, resulting in prostatitis; urethra, resulting in urethritis.

Risk factors for UTI are:

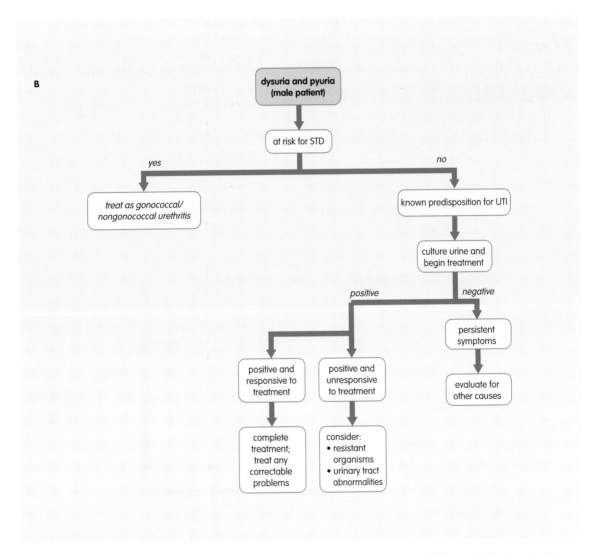

Fig. 6.15 (*Continued*) (B) Dysuria and pyuria in a male patient. STD, sexually transmitted disease; UTI, urinary tract infection (from Green HL 1996 Clinical medicine, 2nd edn. Mosby Year Book).

- Diabetes mellitus.
- Pregnancy.
- Impaired voiding (due to obstruction).
- Genitourinary malformations.
- Sexual intercourse.
- Stones.
- Neurogenic bladder.
- Intact male foreskin.

The main organisms involved are:
- *Escherichia coli* (>70% of cases).
- *Staphylococcus saprophyticus*.
- *Proteus* species.
- *Klebsiella* species.
- *Enterobacter* species.
- *Pseudomonas* species.
- *Enterococcus* species.

 A urinary tract infection in children must always be investigated to exclude vesicoureteric reflux, which can lead to kidney scarring and hypertension.

Diagnostic approach
Algorithms for the investigation of UTI are given in Figs 6.15 and 6.16.

Other presentations of renal disease

Urethral discharge
A urethral discharge is secretion passed through the urethra at times other than voiding. The female equivalent is vaginal discharge. The secretion may be clear, purulent, bloody, itchy or foul smelling.

Causes
Causes of urethral discharge are:
- Non-infectious: irritation (mechanical or chemical), urethral stricture, non-bacterial prostatitis, phimosis, urethral diverticulum, urethral carbuncle. Occasionally, it can be caused by Reiter's syndrome.
- Infectious (i.e. sexually transmitted infections): gonococcal urethritis (characteristically 'canary yellow' discharge) or, more commonly, non-gonococcal urethritis (i.e. *Chlamydia*

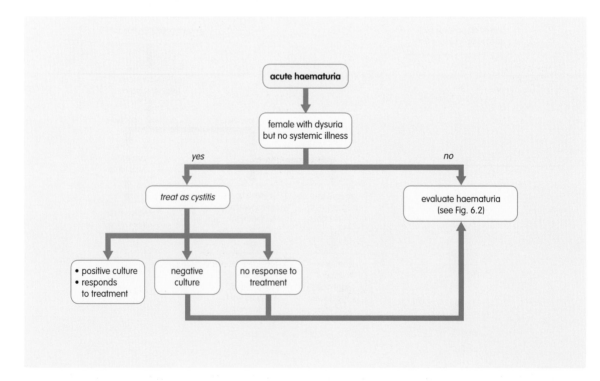

Fig. 6.16 Investigation of urinary tract infection: acute haematuria (from Green HL 1996 Clinical medicine, 2nd edn. Mosby Year Book).

trachomatis, Trichomonas vaginalis, herpes
simplex virus).

Diagnostic approach
An algorithm for diagnosing urethral discharge is
given in Fig. 6.17.

Dysfunctional voiding
In dysfunctional voiding there are abnormal
characteristics of voiding. It is important to find
out how the symptoms differ from normal for
the patient. They can be:

Fig. 6.17 (A) Diagnosing urethral discharge. GNID, Gram-negative intracellular diplococci; GU, gonococcal urethritis;
hpf, high-power field; NGU, non-gonococcal urethritis; PMNs, polymorphonuclear leucocytes (from Green HL 1996
Clinical medicine, 2nd edn. Mosby Year Book).

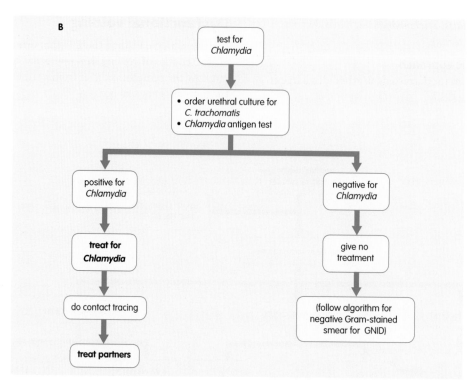

Fig. 6.17 *(Continued)* (B) Investigation for *Chlamydia trachomatis*.

- Irritative: producing frequency, nocturia, urgency and dysuria.
- Obstructive: producing hesitancy, diminished force, dribbling and increased residual urine.

Causes

Irritative bladder symptoms can be caused by:

- Local abnormality with decreased bladder capacity: this can be the result of infection, inflammation or fibrosis. Causes include acute pyogenic infections, chronic infections (i.e. tuberculosis), chlamydia, chronic fungi, foreign body, stones, trauma, radiation, cyclophosphamide, interstitial cystitis and chronic obstruction.
- Neurological abnormality: this can be the result of stroke, cerebral atrophy or multiple sclerosis, all of which damage the cortex or upper spinal cord.

Obstructive bladder symptoms are more common in men because they have a longer urethra, which is easily compressed or narrowed. Causes are summarized in Fig. 6.18.

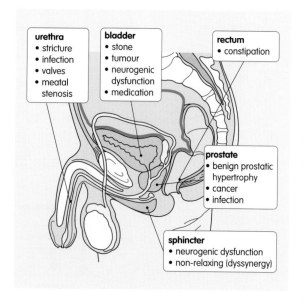

Fig. 6.18 Causes of obstructive bladder symptoms.

Diagnostic approach

A comparison of the aetiology of irritative and obstructive bladder symptoms in dysfunctional voiding is shown in Fig. 6.19.

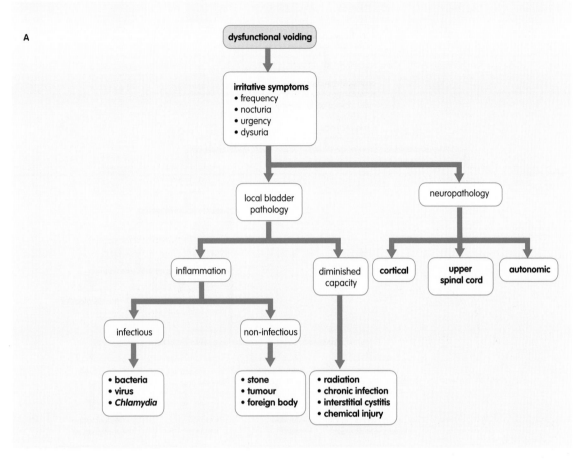

Fig. 6.19 (A) Causes of irritative symptoms in dysfunctional voiding (from Green HL 1996 Clinical medicine, 2nd edn. Mosby Year Book).

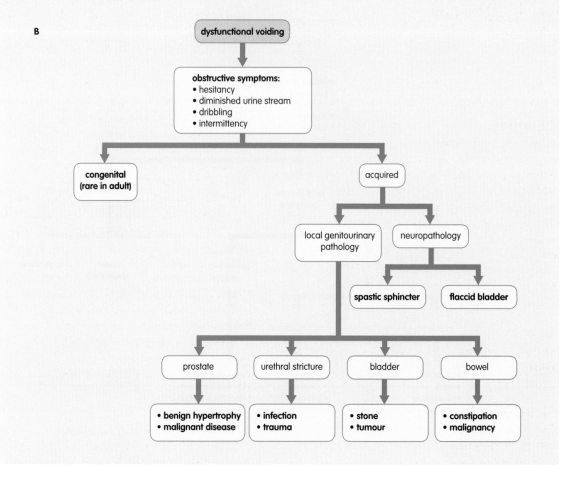

Fig. 6.19 (*Continued*) (B) Causes of obstructive bladder symptoms in dysfunctional voiding (from Green HL 1996 Clinical medicine, 2nd edn. Mosby Year Book).

- Explain the difference between frequency and urgency.
- Describe briefly what urinalysis shows, and what the possible diagnoses are.
- Explain what pseudohyponatraemia is and how it is diagnosed.
- Describe the effect of tissue necrosis on total body K^+, and why this must be corrected urgently.
- List the main causes of ARF, outlining how they are classified.
- Name and define five types of incontinence. Discuss the risk factors for developing incontinence.
- Outline the risk factors for developing a urinary tract infection. Explain why investigation is particularly important in children.
- Explain why *E. coli* and *S. saprophyticus* are the most common organisms to cause urinary tract infections.
- Summarize the defining features of nephrotic syndrome. Describe how primary nephrotic syndrome differs from secondary nephrotic syndrome.
- Outline the tests required to identify chlamydia in a patient presenting with urethral discharge.
- List the three principles of treating patients with sexually transmitted infections.

7. History and Examination

Taking a history

Overview

A full history is essential because it is the first and most important step in making the correct diagnosis. Before taking a history, always introduce yourself—shake hands and tell the patient your name and status (i.e. medical student). Explain what you are going to do and make sure that the patient understands. Before you start, check that the patient is comfortable and relaxed.

Stand back and look around the bedside for clues such as inhalers, oxygen mask, dialysis equipment, blood glucose BM sticks, walking sticks and frames (indicates restricted mobility), sputum pot, cards from the family (show support), and reading material. Also, observe the patient—look for any agitation, difficulties in breathing, speech problems, tremors, deafness.

Structure of the history

The following is a basic guide to structuring the history. Start by taking the patient's name, date of birth and occupation.

Presenting complaint

Allow the patient to explain in his or her own words what the problem is and record the symptoms that the patient describes.

History of the presenting complaint

Features of the presenting complaint to ask about include:

- What is the nature of the complaint? Find out about the symptom, e.g. for pain ask about site, radiation, severity, timing, character (stabbing, burning, pricking), aggravating or relieving factors, and associated symptoms.
- What is the onset and time-course of the complaint? Did the symptom occur gradually or suddenly? When did it begin? Is there a pattern and, if so, what? Find out whether the symptom is intermittent or constant, how frequently it occurs, how long it lasts for and its intensity.
- Are there any precipitating or relieving factors? Does anything bring it on, make it worse or better

(e.g. position, food, pain killers)? In renal colic, the patient will not be comfortable in any position and is constantly moving and writhing.
- Are there other relevant or associated symptoms, e.g. if the presenting complaint is loin pain, ask about urinary frequency, haematuria, nausea or vomiting, constipation or diarrhoea.
- Has the patient had any previous treatment or investigations for this complaint? Has the patient had a similar problem before and what was done about it?

Symptoms relevant to the urinary system are:
- Haematuria (cancer of the renal tract, urinary tract infection, glomerulonephritis).
- Increased frequency (urinary tract infection).
- Poor stream (bladder outflow obstruction—prostatic hypertrophy).
- Nocturia (chronic renal failure or bladder outflow obstruction).

Past medical history

Find out about any illnesses, operations, investigations and treatments, with dates. Elicit the details of past or current medical conditions, such as tuberculosis, asthma, heart conditions, previous strokes, jaundice, epilepsy. Ask about medical conditions associated with renal disease (e.g. diabetes mellitus, hypertension, chronic inflammatory disease, cancer, urinary tract infections, rheumatic fever, tonsillitis, previous renal disease). Make a note of any recent infections—in particular, streptococcal throat infections, as this can trigger postinfective glomerulonephritis.

Obstetric and gynaecological history

Ask about any prolonged labour (resulting in lax pelvic floor muscles), caesarean sections or pelvic inflammatory disease.

Drug history

Determine if the patient:
- Is taking any medications—ask about prescribed and over-the-counter drugs.
- Has any known allergies (e.g. penicillin).
- Has been exposed to any toxins (e.g. industrial toxins, lead, hydrocarbons).

Family history

Note any known medical conditions in first-degree relatives—in particular, renal disease, hypertension and diabetes. Draw a concise diagram of the family tree.

Social history

It is also important to find out the patient's social circumstances. Enquire about the patient's:

- Marital status: children and spouse's health.
- Occupation: current job or past job, effect of illness on job, financial problems.
- Accommodation: where does the patient live and who with? Are there any relatives or friends visiting? Can the patient cope at home (i.e. cooking, washing, home surroundings)?
- Diet and exercise.
- Travel: has the patient been abroad recently?
- Alcohol: how many units does the patient drink? (the best way to assess this is to go through the weekly consumption with the patient).
- Smoking: how much? When did the patient start? If they are an ex-smoker, establish how many years they smoked, how many a day and for how long they have given up.
- Drugs: 'recreational' drugs—how much? How often? For how long?
- Sexual practices.

Systems review

This is a brief overview of all the body systems (Fig. 7.1).

Summary

Always end with a short summary including:

- The name, age and occupation of the patient.
- The presenting complaint and its duration.
- Any relevant associated symptoms or medical history.

Always ask about occupation as patients exposed to carcinogens may develop or worsen existing renal disease.

Communication skills

Effective doctor–patient communication is the basis of accurate history taking, correct diagnosis and successful management. As well as improving the

Brief overview of the body systems	
General/ body system	**Examination**
general questions	weight loss (carcinoma) appetite night sweats fevers (infections) lumps (carcinoma) fatigue (carcinoma)
cardiorespiratory	chest pain (heart disease) dyspnoea palpitations (heart disease) paroxysmal nocturnal dyspnoea ankle oedema (Na^+ and water retention) cough and sputum haemoptysis wheeze (asthma)
gastrointestinal	abdominal pain nausea and vomiting (uraemia) bowel frequency tenesmus or urgency malaena (carcinoma) haematemesis flatulence dysphagia
genitourinary	incontinence* dysuria* haematuria* nocturia* frequency* polyuria* hesitancy* dribbling* menstrual history (cycle and duration, regularity, first day of last menstrual period, number of pregnancies, menarche and menopause)
neurological	fits, blackouts* headaches* sphincter disturbances* dizziness*
musculoskeletal and skin	pain swelling of joints gout rashes/skin conditions*

Fig. 7.1 Summary of systems review. *Asterisks indicate those examinations especially relevant to the renal and urinary systems.

patient's experience of medical care, it offers reassurance and can reduce anxiety. Poor communication can lead to poor compliance, dissatisfaction and mistrust. Ideas and understanding about illness and its implications can vary according to the patient's background and beliefs, so it is important to establish these and develop a care plan that accommodates the patient's needs. Often, a third party will be involved in the patient's care, for example:

- Elderly patients: with their carers.
- Children: with their parents.
- Patients from a different ethnic background: with an interpreter (possibly another family member).
- Patients who are deaf or blind: with an interpreter.

In these cases, clear questioning and explanations are critical to ensure both the patient and the accompanying third party understand what is happening.

When taking a history or examination, always consider the following points:

- Structure the consultation in a logical manner, modifying it to accommodate the patient's needs.
- Appear confident and at ease to reassure the patient. Over 60% of communication is non-verbal, so factors such as posture and eye contact have a significant role in conveying your feelings to the patient.
- Position yourself so you sit facing the patient at the same level. This implies equality—never treat the patient as inferior to you.
- Start with open questions, and then ask closed questions to obtain specific answers. Find out the patient's understanding of the nature of the problem, and his or her perception of what treatment will involve.
- Listen actively and encourage the patient to talk. Actions such as nodding, smiling or echoing the patient's last sentence can help him or her to relax and shows that you are listening. This in turn can prompt the patient to expand on points.
- Allow pauses to encourage the patient to talk further, and to digest what is being said.
- Respond to any concerns that the patient might have and check that the patient understands what is going to happen next.
- Avoid jargon or technical language.
- At the end of the consultation, repeat what the patient has told you to check that you have obtained the correct information, and to clarify any points.

Patient care also involves liaising between many different hospital and community healthcare workers, which again depends on clear communication between these groups.

- Use open questions to establish the patient's beliefs.
- Use closed questions to obtain and classify facts to narrow down the patient's diagnosis.

General inspection

Overview

As stated for taking a medical history, whenever you examine a patient it is very important to remember the following points:

- Always introduce yourself to the patient.
- Observe the patient carefully before you begin the examination, to gain an overall impression of the patient's condition.
- Look around the patient for any extra clues—dialysis equipment, sputum pot or oxygen mask.
- Position the patient appropriately for the examination—at 45 degrees for cardiovascular or respiratory system examination or lying flat for abdominal examination.
- Expose the appropriate part of body only and ensure the patient is comfortable.
- Observe the patient from the end of the bed before you start the examination.
- Notice if the patient is conscious or looks well, is in pain, appears anxious or depressed, smells of urine or has any obvious skeletal abnormalities.
- Look at the patient's stature (Fig. 7.2), any obvious skin pigmentation (Fig. 7.3) and fat distribution.
- The fluid status of the patient should be noted. Useful physical signs include:
  (i) elevated jugular venous pressure (JVP)
  (ii) pleural effusion
  (iii) pulmonary oedema
  (iv) peripheral pitting oedema (most prominent at the ankles and sacrum).
- Signs indicating that the patient is on dialysis include the presence of a dialysis machine, fistula or continuous ambulatory peritoneal dialysis catheter. These indicate that the patient is in acute or end stage renal failure, treated by dialysis.

Face and neck signs related to renal disease are listed in Fig. 7.4.

Fig. 7.2 Signs related to stature and weight in renal disease. BMI body mass index; CRF, chronic renal failure.

Signs related to stature and weight in renal disease		
Test	**Sign**	**Diagnostic inference**
stature	short stature	seen in patients who had CRF in childhood: growth is impaired due to an abnormal response to growth hormone and puberty is delayed
weight and height • measure weight and height • compare with ideal weight for height and calculate body mass index (BMI)	BMI = weight ÷ (height)^2 • underweight if BMI <19 kg/m^2 • obese if BMI >30 kg/m^2 an increase in weight can be due to oedema	• oedema of nephrotic syndrome can be confused with obesity • a low BMI is seen in CRF due to anorexia and malnutrition
oedema (tissue swelling due to accumulation of excess fluid)	• periorbital oedema (swelling of the eyelid) • general puffiness of the face • oedema of the legs • sacral oedema • ascites	renal causes of oedema: • acute glomerulonephritis • nephrotic syndrome • renal failure

Signs related to skin colour in renal disease		
Test	**Sign**	**Diagnostic inference**
pallor	conjunctivae are pale	in CRF, there is a decrease in erythropoietin causing an anaemia with normal iron concentration; other causes of anaemia are iron, vitamin B$_{12}$, and folate deficiency
bruising	areas of skin that are blue/black in colour	in CRF, the bleeding time is increased, leading to bleeding in tissues
pigmentation	areas of darkened skin on either the face or limbs; pale yellow tinge to skin	increased production of melanin-stimulating hormone causes melanin deposition in the skin; also, urochrome deposition in the skin

Fig. 7.3 Signs related to skin colour in renal disease. CRF, chronic renal failure.

Hands and limbs

Abnormalities of the nails that indicate underlying renal disease are summarized in Fig. 7.5. To examine the hands, spread out the fingers on a flat, white surface. This will highlight any shortening of the distal phalanges; a difference of length between the fingers is often seen in severe renal osteodystrophy secondary to chronic renal failure. This is due to chronic high circulating levels of parathyroid hormone. The patient should then hold the hands straight out to the front. Watch for any movement—this can be detected more easily by putting a piece of paper on top of the hands. If a coarse 'dipping' movement is noted in the outstretched fingers, which is exaggerated by wrist dorsiflexion, the possible diagnosis is severe uraemia, a preterminal

Fig. 7.4 Signs in the face and neck related to renal disease. CRF, chronic renal failure; JVP, jugular venous pressure; MSH, melanin-stimulating hormone.

Signs in the face & neck related to renal disease		
Test	**Sign**	**Diagnostic inference**
polycythaemia	red and rugged appearance of the face	occasionally seen in: • polycystic kidneys • post-transplant • carcinoma of the kidney
uraemic frost	white powdery crystals of urate look like dandruff on the forehead	the crystals form from excess urea in the sweat and are a terminal sign of CRF
deposits in the sclera	yellow deposits in the sclera	calcium deposits due to hyperparathyroidism
retinal changes		seen in: • diabetes mellitus • hypertension • vascular disease
ear function	deafness	Alport syndrome
ulcers	ulceration of the mouth and lips	severely ill patients (impaired immune system)
fungal infection	white deposit in the mouth	patients on cytotoxic drugs or steroids; immunosuppression with drugs can result in opportunistic infections such as candidal infection
halitosis (bad breath)	• ammonia smell • acetone smell	• renal failure • ketoacidosis

Nail signs in renal disease		
Test	**Sign**	**Diagnostic inference**
markings on nail	transverse ridges (Beau's lines)	indicative of: • past malnutrition • severe illness
	splinter haemorrhages	renal failure due to: • vasculitis (e.g. Wegener's granulomatosis) • bacterial endocarditis
discoloration of nails	brown discoloration of nails	CRF
	opaque white discoloration of the nails	nephrotic syndrome and CRF

Fig. 7.5 Nail signs in renal disease. CRF, chronic renal failure.

Changes in the limbs in renal disease		
Test	**Sign**	**Diagnostic inference**
appearance and texture of skin	dry flaky skin	CRF
	scratch marks and bruises on limbs and abdomen	uraemic pruritus due to hyperphosphataemia and dry skin
	dirty brown appearance which can make the patient look very healthy or tanned	CRF causing an increase in photosensitive pigment (pseudoporphyrin) as a result of decreased clearance of porphyrins in the urine and increased melanin secondary to increased MSH
skin scars or lesions	fistulae are often seen on the forearm	allow access to blood at a high pressure for haemodialysis
	scars from previous surgically constructed fistulae	vascular access clots and often needs reconstruction
deformities of bones and joints; check range of movement, signs of inflammation and for any pain	valgus (knock knees) and varus (bow legs) deformities	renal rickets due to renal osteodystrophy
	painful, inflamed and red	acute gout due to the deposition of urate crystals in joints
look for any involuntary movement	sporadic twitching of limbs (often accompanies a tremor)	indicative of need for immediate renal replacement therapy
	some patients have an uncontrollable need to move their limbs all the time (restless limbs)	CRF or on dialysis
measure blood pressure	postural drop in BP	hypovolaemia
oedema: pitting if there is indentation of the skin after 10 s of finger pressure	generalized swelling of limb and pitting; if present at ankle, check at knee and mid-thigh	pitting oedema is characteristic of: • fluid overload due to salt and water retention • nephrotic syndrome • congestive cardiac failure
rash	purpuric rash (cutaneous haemorrhage)	vasculitis (e.g. Henoch–Schönlein purpura)
skin and subcutaneous tissue turgor: assessed by rolling a pinch of soft tissue between finger and thumb	the skin will seem less elastic and tense	skin and subcutaneous turgor is reduced in: • old age • Na$^+$ depletion • malnutrition
peripheral neuropathy	a glove and stocking distribution of peripheral sensory loss	advanced renal failure (rare)

Fig. 7.6 Changes in the limbs in renal disease. CRF, chronic renal failure.

sign in patients with renal disease that indicates the need for immediate dialysis.

However, this cannot be distinguished from any of the other metabolic flaps (asterixis) caused by:
• CO_2 retention in respiratory failure.
• Chronic liver disease.

Changes in the limbs in renal disease are listed in Fig. 7.6.

Thorax

Respiratory system

Very few signs in a respiratory examination indicate renal disease. The key change to watch for is the pattern and rate of respiration—patients with a metabolic acidosis associated with chronic renal failure often have a deep, sigh-like respiration, with a rapid breathing rate. This is known as Kussmaul's respiration, and is caused by direct

General findings in the cardiovascular system in renal disease		
Test	**Sign**	**Diagnostic inference**
abnormality of chest wall	increased curvature of spine and rounded shoulders	softening of vertebrae due to renal osteodystrophy in the spine (rugger jersey spine on radiograph)
scars: note position on chest and check round to back following the ribs	midline scars old scars are white and pale and recent scars are purple–red in colour	previous heart surgery
jugular venous pressure (an indicator of internal fluid load): the patient should be at 45° and with head turned away from you; note any pulsations in the internal jugular vein	normally jugular venous pulse is not visible, but can be seen by occluding the vein just above the clavicle if a waveform is visible then measure the height from the top of the fluid level vertically down to the angle of Louis	jugular venous pressure is raised in: • right heart failure • fluid overload • chronic bronchitis

Fig. 7.7 Superficial findings in the cardiovascular system in renal disease.

stimulation of the respiratory centre in an attempt to correct the systemic acidosis. A similar respiratory pattern is seen in severe untreated diabetic ketoacidosis.

Cardiovascular system (CVS)
Blood pressure (BP)
Many patients with renal disease will have an elevated BP. When measuring BP (which needs to be done on several occasions) it is important to measure it on the same limb each time to ensure consistent and comparable results. To ensure measurement is accurate:
• Select the correct cuff size.
• Use the cuff on a fully extended arm with the stethoscope applied lightly to the brachial artery.
• Always take the BP with the patient lying, sitting and standing. This is because a 5–10mmHg increase in diastolic pressure is usually seen on standing in a healthy CVS. Postural hypotension (i.e. a drop in diastolic pressure on standing) can be detected only if both measurements are made.

The World Health Organization (WHO) defines hypertension as a maintained systolic pressure of 140mmHg or above and a diastolic pressure of 90mmHg or above. Renal diseases associated with hypertension include renal artery stenosis, acute and chronic glomerulonephritis (GN), polycystic kidneys, and nephrotic syndrome.

Observation, palpation, percussion and auscultation
Examine the CVS with the patient sitting at 45° and undressed from the waist up. Figure 7.7 summarizes the superficial signs in the CVS in renal disease and Fig. 7.8 shows the findings on palpation in the CVS examination. Percussion of the heart borders can be dull beyond the normal boundaries of the mediastinum, which suggests an enlarged heart. Decreased breath sounds at the bases of the lungs indicates a pleural effusion, which can occur in:
• Nephrotic syndrome.
• Congestive heart failure.
• Fluid retention.

The positive findings on auscultation of the CVS are shown in Fig. 7.9.

Abdomen

Overview
The patient should be lying as flat as possible on a firm mattress with arms by the side and head supported with one or two pillows—check that the patient is comfortable. This position ensures that the abdominal muscles are relaxed, making palpation much easier.

Stand on the right hand side of the bed, ideally with the patient exposed from 'nipples to knees'; to maintain privacy expose the patient from the xiphisternum to the level of the symphysis pubis.

Findings on palpation in the cardiovascular system examination in renal disease

Test	Sign	Diagnostic inference
apex beat is normally felt in the mid-clavicular line at the level of the fifth intercostal space; this is the most lateral point at which the pulsation can be felt—note its position and strength	lateral displacement	left ventricular dilatation causing enlargement of the heart pneumothorax
	impalpable	• obesity • pleural effusion • pericardial effusion
	thrusting and strong	• high blood pressure • left ventricular hypertrophy
peripheral pulses	presence or absence listen with a stethoscope for bruits	atherosclerosis if present may suggest renovascular disease

Fig. 7.8 Findings on palpation of the cardiovascular system in renal disease.

Positive findings on auscultation of the cardiovascular system in renal disease

Test	Sign	Diagnostic inference
heart sounds: listen for audibility, rate and accentuation of the sound in all four areas	muffled and soft	pericardial effusion
	prominent aortic component of the second heart sound	hypertension
	a low-pitched third heart sound heard after the second heart sound	an early sign of left ventricular failure or fluid overload
	gallop rhythm (two normal heart sounds with a third and tachycardia)	• fluid overload • ventricular failure
murmurs: • low pitch (apex) with the bell • high pitch with the diaphragm feel the carotid pulse—time the murmur with the cardiac cycle	• functional murmurs • murmurs due to coexisting valve disease	• aortic and pulmonary regurgitation due to dilatation of the valve ring secondary to fluid overload • mitral regurgitation due to annular calification of the valve; anaemia
pericardial rub: listen carefully over the precordium	a localized or generalized scratchy sound heard in any part of the cardiac cycle heard best if the patient leans forward	this friction rub (two layers of the pericardial layer moving in the presence of an exudate) occurs in: • pericarditis (a terminal feature of CRF) • uraemic pericarditis • systemic lupus erythematosus and vasculitis • intermittent illness in a patient with CRF

Fig. 7.9 Auscultatory findings of the cardiovascular system in renal disease. CRF, chronic renal failure.

Examination of the genitalia is a vital part of examination of the abdominal system. They should either be covered up once inspection is complete or be examined later. Remember to tell the patient that you will need to examine the genitalia and to perform a rectal examination and (if the patient is female) vaginal examination.

Inspection

Spend the first 20–30s inspecting the patient from the end of the bed. Look around the patient for any clues—drips, drains and dialysis machines. Figure 7.10 shows the signs usually seen on general inspection of the abdomen in a patient with renal disease.

	Signs on general inspection of the abdomen in renal disease	
Test	**Sign**	**Diagnostic inference**
abnormality of the abdominal contours: • general distension	• general fullness and enlargement of the abdominal cavity • the skin of the abdomen is shiny and smooth	renal causes of a distended abdomen are: • fluid (ascites or CAPD fluid) other (nonrenal) causes include: • fat • flatus • fetus • faeces (constipation)
• localized distension observe to see if abdomen moves with or independently of respiration	symmetrical swelling	polycystic kidneys
	asymmetrical swelling	enlarged kidney; kidney transplant in the iliac regions
scars: note position on the abdomen and check round to the back following the ribs to the spine	midline scars	previous abdominal surgery
	iliac scars overlying a mass	kidney transplants
	lateral longitudinal scars extending around the back	nephrectomy scars
	note that old scars are white and pale and recent scars are purple–red in colour	

Fig. 7.10 Findings on general inspection of the abdomen in renal disease. CAPD, continuous ambulatory peritoneal dialysis.

Palpation

Before palpating, check if the patient is in pain. If the answer is yes, ask where the painful or tender area is and start palpating from the point furthest from the locus of the pain. Tell the patient to breathe normally and relax—you will be able to feel much more through relaxed abdominal muscles. It can help to kneel at the bedside so that you are at the same level as the patient—always demonstrate this in an examination.

Develop a routine for examining all the regions and organs to avoid omitting anything:

- Begin with gentle palpation of the nine regions of the abdomen; then repeat using deeper palpation—keep looking at the patient's face for any signs of discomfort.
- Feel for the liver and spleen while the patient is breathing deeply in and out.
- Next examine the kidneys and urinary bladder, feeling for the aorta, and then check the hernial orifices (inguinal and femoral) while the patient is coughing.

- If you feel a mass, define its site, size, shape, edge, surface (regular or irregular), consistency, mobility, movement with respiration and whether it is pulsatile or resonant to percussion. Also check for associated scars and listen over the mass for a bruit.
- Remember to tell the patient that you need to examine the genitalia and to perform a digital rectal examination (see p. 151).

Figure 7.11 explains how the kidneys are examined and shows relevant findings in various renal conditions. The differentiating features between an enlarged left kidney and splenomegaly are summarised in Fig. 7.12.

Beware! An enlarged kidney can easily be confused with:
- Hepatomegaly (right).
- Splenomegaly (left).

How the kidneys are examined and relevant findings in various renal conditions		
Test	**Sign**	**Diagnostic inference**
bimanual examination of the kidneys: • place the right hand anteriorly in the lumbar region and the left hand posteriorly under the patient in the loin • push up with the left hand as the patient takes a deep breath in • ballot the kidneys between both hands (i.e. push the kidney from one hand to the other) • repeat on the other side keeping the right hand anterior	the kidney is normally impalpable (except in very thin people) and if easily felt suggests an abnormality the lower pole is felt as a firm round edge between both hands on deep inspiration (it must be distinguished from an enlarged liver or spleen) there is minimal movement on respiration an irregular kidney surface felt in polycystic disease	unilateral enlargement: • tumour • renal cyst • hydronephrosis • compensatory hypertrophy bilateral enlargement: • polycystic kidneys • hydronephrosis • tumour (rare)
examination of the urinary bladder: • the bladder is palpated from the umbilicus down to the symphysis pubis • the upper and lateral borders are easily felt • the inferior border is impalpable	not normally palpable when enlarged it is felt as a smooth rounded firm cystic mass in the suprapubic region it is not always symmetrical and in the midline	chronic retention of urine acute retention is associated with bladder tenderness distended bladders are not always palpable in obesity
pain: • check carefully if the patient is in pain • the nature of the pain is important in determining the site of the lesion • assess pain by asking the patient to point to the pain and asking what the pain is like	fixed constant pain; colicky pain superimposed on a constant dull pain	kidney pain
	radiation of pain from the flank to the groin and iliac fossa; the patient is usually writhing in pain and is doubled up	ureteric distension due to obstruction in the ureters, most commonly renal stones as they are passed down the ureter

Fig. 7.11 How to examine the kidneys and relevant findings in a variety of renal conditions.

Distinguishing features differentiating left kidney enlargement and splenomegaly	
Enlarged left kidney	**Splenomegaly**
moves late with inspiration	moves early in inspiration
can feel above it	cannot get above it; enlarges towards the umbilicus
smooth surface	notched border palpable
resonant to percussion	dull to percussion

Fig 7.12 Distinguishing factors between left kidney enlargement and splenomegaly.

Percussion

Percussion in the abdomen is used to elicit the cause of any distension and the composition of any mass—fluid-filled cysts and solid tumours are dull to percussion. Figure 7.13 shows the findings observed on percussion of the abdomen in patients with renal disease.

 Remember the causes of a distended abdomen as the 5 Fs:
• Fat.
• Fluid.
• Flatus.
• Fetus.
• Faeces.

Findings observed on percussion of the abdomen in renal disease		
Test	**Sign**	**Diagnostic inference**
ascites (excess free fluid in the peritoneal cavity): • presence shown by shifting of dullness • the abdomen is percussed from the flank into the midline for any areas of dullness • keep your hand on the area of dullness • ask the patient to roll away from you on to his or her side • percuss in this area with the patient in the new position and see if it is now resonant to percussion • this can be confirmed by asking the patient to roll over onto the other side	positive shifting dullness is indicative of ascites the area that was previously dull to percussion becomes resonant due to redistribution of fluid in the peritoneal cavity	causes of ascites in renal disease: • nephrotic syndrome • peritoneal dialysis • idiopathic ascites of dialysis • perineal dialysis fluid
percussion of the bladder: always percuss from above the umbilicus down to the pubic bone	resonance followed by dullness consistent with an enlarged cystic mass	distension of the urinary bladder due to chronic or acute retention

Fig. 7.13 Findings on percussion of the abdomen in renal disease.

Prostate findings on digital rectal examination	
Sign	**Diagnostic inference**
firm, smooth, rubbery consistency; walnut-shaped and sized	normal prostate
tender, enlarged and soft	acute infection (prostatitis)
hard, irregular, asymmetric, nodular	prostate carcinoma

Fig. 7.14 Changes of the prostate noted on digital rectal examination.

Auscultation

Auscultate for bruits by applying the stethoscope firmly on the abdomen or in the flank over the renal artery. Alternatively, they can be heard over the back. However, it can be difficult to distinguish an aortic bruit from one originating in the renal artery. A bruit is heard if there is rapid turbulent movement of blood through a narrowed artery. Causes of bruits include:
• Renal artery stenosis.
• Atherosclerosis.
• Arteriovenous malformation in the kidney.

Digital rectal examination (DRE)

Always obtain permission and have a chaperone for female patients. The patient should lie on the left side, with the knees drawn up to the chest.
• Inspect the perianal area for haemorrhoids, fissures, inflammation, prolapse and ulcers.
• Put lubricant on the glove and insert finger into the rectum.
• Assess the tone of the anal sphincter, the size and shape of the prostate (normally walnut sized).
• After removing your finger, inspect for any blood or faeces.
• Feel for any lateral masses.

Palpable changes in the prostate and their clinical significance are summarized in Fig. 7.14. A vaginal examination should also be performed in female patients.

- Describe which symptoms are particularly relevant to the urinary system.
- Briefly describe the skills required to conduct an effective consultation.
- List what you might see around a patient to help you assess the patient's condition.
- Describe the skin changes associated with renal disease.
- Describe the two main differentials if a patient is admitted with a rapid sigh-like deep respiration. Outline the signs and symptoms that might help you differentiate between them.
- Explain how you can ensure that blood pressure (BP) measurement is consistent and comparable. Discuss why it is important to measure BP lying, sitting and standing.
- List the possible findings on auscultation of the heart in renal disease.
- Describe how to examine the kidneys. List the possible causes for unilateral and bilateral kidney enlargement.
- Explain how you can test for ascites, and what the renal-related causes are.
- Outline the possible findings on digital rectal examination.

8. Investigation and Imaging

When considering investigations, always start with the least invasive simple procedures and then progress to second-line investigations if required.

To take an MSU:
- The patient must have a full bladder.
- Clean the external urethral meatus with a sterile swab.
- Collect the sample half way through urine flow.

Testing the blood and urine

Renal and urinary tract diseases are indicated if the patient presents with symptoms linked to the urinary tract, abnormal serum urea or creatinine concentration, or abnormal urinalysis. Testing the urine is the simplest investigation and should always be done in suspected renal disease. This is done with a midstream urine sample, and assessment includes appearance, volume, pH, dipstick, microscopy and cytology (Figs 8.1 and 8.2).

Blood tests that assess the basic renal function include plasma urea and creatinine. However, a significant amount of renal damage can occur before abnormal values are detected in the blood, so the preferred option is to measure creatinine clearance,

Microbiological test results and their significance				
	Indications	Scientific basis	Normal results	Abnormal results
urine culture	must always be performed if UTI symptoms or any renal disease is suspected; in cases of TB an early morning sample of urine is required	growing any organisms present; vital to have an MSU specimen	no growth	>100 000 CFU/mL indicates urinary infection < 10 000 CFU/mL probably indicates contamination of the specimen
antibodies (i) streptococcal Ag	suspicion of past streptococcal glomerulonephritis	antibodies are made in response to infection and may trigger glomerulonephritis		increased titres of: AntiDNAase B ASOT consistent with poststreptococcal glomerulonephrits
(ii) hepatitis	renal disease associated with liver disease	infection with hepatits B and C have effects on the kidney		hepatitis B causes polyarteritis nodosa membranous nephropathy hepatitis C causes cryoglobulinaemia
(iii) HIV	patients at risk of HIV with renal symptoms	infection with HIV can cause renal damage		HIV-associated glomerulonephritis
malaria	those who have recently returned from the tropics and have recurrent fevers			ring-form parasites observed on peripheral blood film

Fig. 8.1 Microbiological tests and their significance. Ag, antigen; ASOT, antistreptococcal O antigen titre; CFU, colony-forming units; HIV, human immunodeficiency virus; MSU, midstream urine.

which closely reflects the GFR (see Chapter 1). A full blood count highlights anaemia (due to blood loss or impaired renal function) and polycythaemia (raised urate levels). Other important blood results are shown in Fig. 8.3.

Imaging and other investigations

Imaging is a very useful investigation in renal disease when used in conjunction with other investigative techniques. Radiological imaging of the upper and lower urinary tract can be used to:

- Establish a diagnosis.
- Assess the complications of impaired renal function.
- Monitor the progression of disease.
- Follow the response to treatment.

> - Imaging of the upper urinary tract includes KUB radiography, ultrasonography, CT and IVU.
> - The main form of imaging for the lower urinary tract is cystoscopy.

Plain radiography

Plain radiography of the kidney, ureters and bladder (KUB) is a simple, non-invasive test that can be used before specialized imaging. It is used to detect calcification in the kidney, such as renal and urinary tract stones—uric acid stones cannot be detected, but in general 90% of stones are radio-opaque (Figs 8.4 and 8.5). It also highlights the size and position of the kidneys, and any bony deposits (these can be associated with prostatic cancer).

> The main type of radiograph used to visualize the renal system and urinary tract is a KUB—NOT a plain abdominal view, as this often does not include the full pelvis.

Ultrasonography

Ultrasonography is another non-invasive technique that involves high frequency sound waves. It is used to assess the size, shape and position of the kidney, and can also distinguish solid masses and renal cysts (Figs 8.6 and 8.7). Dilatation of the pelvicalyceal system and upper ureters can also be detected—indicating the presence of obstruction. This is a major cause of reversible renal failure, and can be treated if detected early enough. Prostate size can also be assessed, and if necessary, a biopsy can be taken under transurethral ultrasonography guidance for further investigation (Fig. 8.8). Renal vein thrombosis can be detected with Doppler ultrasonography, and arterial Doppler studies can be used to identify renal artery stenosis. The specificity and sensitivity of ultrasound investigations are very operator dependent.

Renal biopsy

Renal biopsy is used for the histological classification of glomerulonephritis, as this can influence the choice of therapy in patients with nephrotic syndrome and acute nephritis. It is also used in the diagnosis and assessment of systemic diseases that affect the kidneys, e.g. sarcoidosis, SLE. It can aid the investigation of unexplained acute renal failure, proteinuria, and haematuria and is vital in the management of renal transplant patients. A sample of the kidney tissue can be taken by inserting a needle into the back using ultrasound guidance, with the patient lying in the prone position. This is then examined under a microscope, using immunochemical staining to detect complement or immunoglobulins. Relative contraindications to renal biopsy include:

- A bleeding diathesis (absolute unless corrected).
- Single kidney (risk of loss).
- Obesity (technically difficult).
- Small kidneys (technically difficult).
- Pregnancy.
- Renal failure (increased risk of bleeding).

The main complications are bleeding (haematuria), infection, pain in the flank and possibly shoulder tip (referred pain) and renal haematoma/scarring.

Intravenous urography and intravenous pyelography

Intravenous urography (IVU) and pyelography (IVP) involve serial radiographs taken after intravenous

Urine biochemistry test results and their significance

	Indications	Scientific basis	Normal results	Abnormal results
appearance	any urine sample		clear fluid	**red/pink:** haematuria, beetroot intake **brown:** concentrated cholestatic jaundice **cloudy:** infection
volume	any urine sample		1000–2500 mL/day	**oliguria:** physiological; intrinsic renal disease; obstructive nephropathy **polyuria:** excess H_2O intake; increased solute loss e.g. glucose; concentration failure
pH	any urine sample		pH 4.5–8.0	**alkaline urine:** infection with *Proteus*—urea splitting **acid urine:** aminoaciduria; renal calculi
sodium	oliguria altered Na^+ homeostasis	urinary [Na] must be interpreted in context of urine output, sodium intake and natriuretic drugs	depends on clinical setting; 24-hour urinary Na^+ = 100–250 mmol/L	<20 mmol/L oligouria minoaciduria; renal calculi <20 mmol/L oligouria →prerenal <20 mmol/L and not oligouric →extrarenal losses >20 mmol/L renal losses
creatinine and creatinine clearance	similar to those for blood creatinine levels	creatinine clearance reflects GFR; both the urine and plasma concentration of creatinine is required; requires timed urine collection	125 mL/min per 1.73 m^2 body surface area	decreased levels indicate a decrease in GFR—as see in acute and chronic renal diseases
blood	gross bleeding into urine usually found in patients with renal disease; hypertension; pregnancy; bacterial endocarditis	reagent strips are used—based on a peroxide-like reaction	nil any positive result must be followed by microscopy	**microscopic haematuria:** renal disease, i.e. nephritic syndrome; blood at the beginning of voiding then clear—from the urethra; blood throughout voiding—from the bladder or above; blood only at the end of voiding—from the prostate or base of the bladder
protein dipstick and if positive → 24-hour collection	oedema	reagent strips impregnated with buffered blue tetrabromophenol—detects [albumin] >150 mg/L; microalbuminuria is used as an earlier indicator of diabetic glomerular disease; the test requires a radioimmunoassay ↑ which is more sensitive than the strips	<150 mg /day random sample = < 100 mg/L (>0.3g/L is detected on the sticks) microalbuminuria = 30–150 μg/min or 0.2–2.8 mg/mmol of protein	**increased with:** exercise; standing up; renal disease; nephrotic syndrome; fever; diabetic glomerular disease; hypertension
glucose	suspected diabetes mellitus; renal disease; pregnancy	reagent strips using glucose oxidase or hexokinase enzyme reactions Clinitest	nil	glucose may be present when: 1. blood glucose above the renal threshold i.e. diabetes mellitus 2. altered renal threshold i.e. pregnancy; renal disease
urine microscopy (obtain a clean urine sample i.e. MSU) (i) direct (ii) after centrifugation	symptoms of UTIs; suspicion of renal disease	a small amount of unspun urine placed on a slide, covered with a cover slip and looked at under a microscope. Gram stain to look for bacteria counterstained to look at cell cytology	nil	**white cells indicate:** inflammatory reaction; infection in the urinary tract; stones; TB; analgesic nephropathy **red cells indicate:** glomrulonephritis; acute urinary tract infection; calculi; tumour **granular casts indicate:** acute tubular necrosis; rapidly progressing glomerulonephritis **white blood cell casts indicate:** pyelonephritis **red cell casts indicate:** glomerulonephritis **crystals seen indicate:** stones **bacteria seen indicate:** infection **abnormal cells indicate:** cancer of urothelium

Fig. 8.2 Urine test results and their significance. MSU, midstream urine; TB, tuberculosis; UTI, urinary tract infection. ESR, erythrocyte sedimentation rate; GFR, glomerular filtration rate; PSA, prostate-specific antigen; UTI, urinary tract infection.

155

Blood test results and their significance				
	Indications	Scientific basis	Normal results	Abnormal results
urea	oligouria & anuria; dehydration; hypertension; diabetes mellitus; oedema; nausea & vomiting; loin pain	crude indication of renal function	2.5–6.6 mmol/L	increased in: renal disease; high protein intake; fever; gastrointestinal haemorrhage
creatinine	same as above for urea	reciprocal relationship with GFR—reflects renal function	62–124 mmol/L	increased in all types of renal disease; N.B. GFR may fall by 50% before urea or creatinine go outside the reference range
albumin	oedema	gives an assessment of severity of urinary protein losses in proteinuria	35–50 g/L	hypoalbuminaemia nephrotic syndome hyperalbuminaemia dehydration
sodium, potassium, anion gap	confusion; lethargy; seizures; coma; arrythmias; hypertension; hypotension; tachycardia/ bradycardia; vomiting; diarrhoea; heavy sweating; diabetes mellitus; polyuria; polydipsia	changes in the concentration of sodium, potassium and the anion gap are found in renal diseases; potassium is important in the function of excitable tissues and is important for survival	Na=135–145 mmol/L K=3.5–5.0 mmol/L anion gap = 8–16 mmol/L	hypernatraemia hyponatraemia hyperkalaemia hypokalaemia increased anion gap in: renal failure ketoacidosis (diabetes melitus) hyperlactaemia (from shock) anion ingestion
arterial blood gases and pH (uses arterial blood)	hypoperfusion; hyperventilation; Kussmaul's breathing in diabetic ketoacidosis; ingestion of acids; diarrhoea; vomiting	oxygen concentration is important as it reflects tissue perfusion; an increase in CO_2 is lethal and poisonous to cells; pH is vital because most cells in the body work at an optimal pH and are very sensitive to changes in pH	pO_2 = 10.6–13.0 kPa pCO_2 = 4.7–6.0 kPa pH = 7.35–7.45	acidosis commonly found in renal failure; compensated for by respiratory stimulation ↓ pCO_2
haemoglobin	chronic renal failure; haemorrhage	the haemoglobin levels are important as Hb carries oxygen to the tissues.	male 13.5–18.0 g/dL female 11.5–16.0 g/dL	decreased Hb chronic renal failure blood loss polycythaemia renal tumours renal cysts
ESR	loin pain; symptoms of UTI; systemic disease		<15 mm/h	increased in infection renal cell carcinoma retroperitoneal fibrosis vasculitis
PSA (prostate-specific antigen)	any men aged >45 years with prostatism or UTIs	the level of PSA increases with prostatic cancer and metastatic disease; used to monitor therapy success		increased in prostatic carcinoma silent recurrence of carcinoma metastatic disease small increase in prostatic hyperplasia
urate	kidney stones; patients with large tumour loads given chemotheraphy; 'tumour lysis' syndrome → urate	hyperuricaemia can cause urate deposition in renal tract	0.12–0.42 mmol/L	increased in gout renal and urinary calculi
calcium	kidney stones; myeloma; metastatic disease	hypercalcaemia causes calcium deposition in renal tract; hypercalcuria also causes urinary concentrating defects	2.0–2.6 mmol/L	increased in renal and urinary calculi

Fig. 8.3 Blood test results and their significance.

156

Fig. 8.4 Plain abdominal radiograph showing several calculi in the left kidney (Courtesy of Mr RS Cole).

Fig. 8.6 Ultrasound scan showing the typical appearance of polycystic kidneys. There are multiple cysts within the parenchyma (from Lloyd-Davis RW et al 1994 Color atlas of urology, 2nd edn. Mosby Year Book).

Fig. 8.5 This plain abdominal radiograph shows a large staghorn calculus in the right kidney in a patient who presented with recurrent urinary tract infections (from Williams G, Mallick NP 1994 Color atlas of renal diseases, 2nd edn. Mosby Year Book).

Fig. 8.7 Hydronephrosis of the right kidney demonstrated by ultrasonography. The echo-lucent (black) areas within the kidney are caused by dilated calyces (from Williams G, Mallick NP 1994 Color atlas of renal diseases, 2nd edn. Mosby Year Book).

injection of radio-opaque contrast medium (Figs 8.9 and 8.10). Normal kidney function is required, and the patient must not be pregnant. These techniques are used to assess kidney size and shape as well as the anatomy and patency of the calyces, pelvis and ureters. It can also be used to localize fistulae and highlight filling defects in the bladder.

When considering investigations involving contrast, always remember that risks of the procedure include allergy to the contrast medium and reaction to the contrast. This ranges from mild (itching, nausea and vomiting) to severe reaction, which could impair renal function—especially if the patient has pre-existing renal disease.

Renal arteriography

Renal arteriography uses contrast medium to give an anatomical demonstration of the renal arteries. It is used to detect renal artery stenosis or aneurysms (Figs 8.11 and 8.12A) and to investigate renal hypertension. Renal artery stenosis can be

Investigation and Imaging

Fig. 8.8 A rectal ultrasound probe is used to define and stage carcinoma of the prostate. The arrow highlights an echo-poor area in the left peripheral zone of the prostate. This extends into the central part of the gland and beyond the capsule (courtesy of Dr D Rickards).

Fig. 8.10 An intravenous urogram showing marked calyceal clubbing in the right kidney. There is gross dilatation of the calyces, which is pronounced in all poles of the kidney. These findings are the result of unilateral reflux of urine and chronic infection (from Lloyd-Davis RW et al 1994 Color atlas of urology, 2nd edn. Mosby Year Book).

Fig. 8.9 An intravenous urogram showing bilateral hydronephrosis in response to bladder neck obstruction caused by dense granulation and fibrous tissue in a patient with schistosomiasis of the bladder (from Williams G, Mallick NP 1994 Color atlas of renal diseases, 2nd edn. Mosby Year Book).

Fig. 8.11 Subtraction arteriogram of a transplanted kidney. The donor renal artery is anastamosed to the internal iliac artery (from Williams G, Mallick NP 1994 Color atlas of renal diseases, 2nd edn. Mosby Year Book).

highlighted using magnetic resonance aided angiography (Fig 8.12B). Therapeutic angioplasty may be performed at the same time. It can be used in the diagnosis of tumours, but this is becoming less common with the increasing use of CT. A catheter is introduced into the femoral artery, through which contrast is injected into the renal artery and a series of radiographs are taken.

Micturating cystourethrography

Micturating cystourethrograms are used to demonstrate vesicoureteric reflux from the bladder to the ureters during emptying of the bladder (Fig. 8.13). Reflux can be classified into three grades.

• Grade 1: contrast medium enters the ureter only.

Fig. 8.13 A micturating cystourethrogram showing bilateral ureteric reflux. This patient has early calyceal clubbing (A) and ureteric dilatation (B). This is grade-3 reflux (courtesy Mr RS Cole).

Fig. 8.12 (A) An arteriogram showing a marked renal arterial stenosis on the right, typical of fibromuscular hyperplasia. (B) MR renal angiography demonstrating a tight stenosis at the origin of the right renal artery. The irregularity of the abdominal aorta is due to marked atheroma.

- Grade 2: contrast medium fills the pelvicalyceal system.
- Grade 3: dilatation of the calyces and ureter.

This technique was used to investigate children with recurrent urinary tract infections but has largely been replaced by other techniques because of concerns over ionizing radiation. It continues to have a role in the investigation of adults with disturbed bladder function.

Cystoscopy

A rigid or flexible cystoscope is inserted through the urethra to inspect the interior surface of the lower urinary tract (bladder and urethra). This technique is very useful in the diagnosis and treatment of tumours in the bladder. It can also be used to identify stones and fistulae, take a tissue biopsy and to assess prostatic disease.

Diagnostic cystoscopy can be performed in the outpatient clinic, and involves a flexible cystoscope examination under local anaesthesia. Therapeutic cystoscopy requires a hospital admission and uses a rigid cystoscope, with the patient under general anaesthesia.

Retrograde pyelography

Retrograde pyelography is used to define the site of an obstruction (Figs 8.14 and 8.15) or lesions within the ureter. It does not require functioning kidneys. The patient must be admitted for general anaesthesia and a ureteric catheter is then inserted under cystoscopic guidance. Contrast medium is injected into the catheter, to identify any lesions and help dislodge ureteric stones and coax them down the ureter.

Fig. 8.14 Retrograde pyelogram showing 'emphysematous' pyelonephritis caused by gas-forming bacteria (from Catto GRD et al 1994 Diagnostic picture tests in renal disease. TMIP).

Fig. 8.16 CT scan highlighting a right renal cell carcinoma that extends through the intercostal space between ribs 11 and 12 (arrow) and medially along the renal vein. The high density (white) areas (arrows) indicate calcification (from Williams G, Mallick NP 1994 Color atlas of renal diseases, 2nd edn. Mosby Year Book).

Fig. 8.15 Retrograde pyelogram showing a large filling defect in the left ureter (arrow) caused by a tumour (from Lloyd-Davis RW et al 1994 Color atlas of urology, 2nd edn. Mosby Year Book).

Antegrade pyelography

This is used to define the site of obstruction in the upper urinary tract, i.e. mainly within the pelvicalyceal system. It involves percutaneous catheterization of a renal calyx and injection of contrast medium as described above for retrograde pyelography. Percutaneous catheterization of the pelvicalyceal system (nephrostomy) is also used therapeutically to relieve obstruction.

Computed tomography (CT)

CT is a quick and non-invasive technique, which can be used with or without contrast. It is used to define renal and retroperitoneal masses and is ideal for locating and staging renal tumours (Fig. 8.16). It is also used to show polycystic kidney disease and has the advantage of also highlighting non-renal pathology. Modern techniques involving spiral CT can be used to visualize the anatomy of the renal arteries, renal vein and inferior vena cava, as well as retroperitoneal studies. Increasingly, CT is the investigation of choice to diagnose obstruction to the urinary tract (Fig. 8.17).

Magnetic resonance imaging (MRI)

MRI is an imaging technique that does not involve ionizing radiation—unlike CT. Instead, it relies on the measurement of the magnetic fields of atomic nuclei. It is used to differentiate between cystic and solid renal masses and for precise staging of tumours. However, MRI is expensive and cannot be used in patients with pacemakers or other metallic implants. Magnetic resonance has now been developed to

Fig. 8.17 An abdominal CT scan of a patient who presented with acute renal failure and bilateral loin pain. There is bilateral hydronephrosis secondary to bilateral ureteric stones. In the upper image a nephrostomy tube is seen in the right renal pelvis. The lower image demonstrates a dense opacity (calculus) lying in the ureter approximately at the level of L2. Subsequent images demonstrated a similar opacity at L3 on the left.

Fig. 8.18 (A) ^{99m}Tc-DMSA scan showing a right upper pole scar (courtesy TO Nunan). (B) The graph shows a diminished uptake of 36% for the right kidney, indicating a degree of loss of function correlating with the scar (from Williams G, Mallick NP 1994 Color atlas of renal diseases, 2nd edn. Mosby Year Book).

provide resolution sufficient to diagnose atheromatous renal artery stenosis (see Fig. 8.12B).

Radionuclide scanning

Radionuclide scans are used in static and dynamic imaging. Technetium-labelled dimercaptosuccinic acid (^{99m}Tc-DMSA) provides static images of the renal parenchyma and shows local renal function. It highlights the localization, shape and function of each individual kidney, and highlights scarring as a result of reflux nephropathy (Fig. 8.18) Technetium-labelled pentetic acid (^{99m}Tc-DTPA) is excreted by renal filtration and the changes in the level of ^{99m}Tc-DTPA in the kidney over time are quantified using a gamma camera. This provides a dynamic index of blood flow to each kidney. It is used to assess transplant function (Fig. 8.19A) and can demonstrate obstruction to the upper urinary tract (by diuresis renogram, Fig. 8.19B). It can also be used to determine the relative function of each kidney. Both ^{99m}Tc-DMSA and ^{99m}Tc-DTPA are injected into the venous circulation. Radionuclide techniques can be used to demonstrate reflux nephropathy.

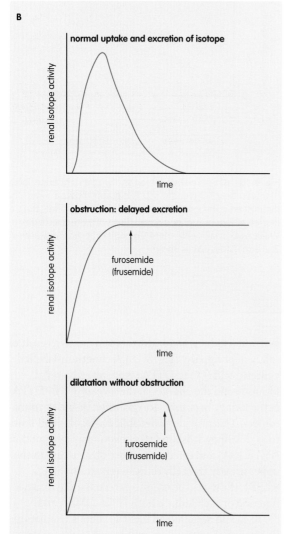

Urodynamic studies

These are used to distinguish urge incontinence from genuine stress incontinence. They also detect bladder/detrusor muscle instability. The bladder is catheterized and a pressure probe is inserted to measure the bladder pressure. A rectal probe is also inserted to assess intra-abdominal pressure. The detrusor muscle pressure can be calculated by subtracting the bladder pressure from the intra-abdominal pressure. The bladder is then filled with water until the patient feels the urge to void. At this point the relative pressures are recorded. If the patient has stress incontinence, an increase in intra-abdominal pressure (e.g. coughing) leads to involuntary urine leakage, with no bladder/detrusor muscle contraction. If the patient has urge incontinence, the bladder/detrusor muscle contracts either spontaneously or with increased abdominal pressure, and the patient feels an overwhelming urge to urinate immediately (Fig. 8.20).

Other imaging techniques

Other imaging techniques include scintigraphy, which is used to investigate vesicoureteric reflux (Fig. 8.21).

Fig. 8.19 (A) ^{99m}Tc-DTPA diuretic renogram showing a transplanted kidney functioning normally (from Catto GRD et al 1994 Diagnostic picture tests in renal disease. TMIP). (B) Diuretic isotopic renography showing tracings for normal, obstructed and dilated (without obstruction) upper urinary tract. Obstruction can be distinguished from dilatation by administering furosemide (frusemide), which promotes excretion of the isotope in dilatation (without obstruction) but has no effect on excretion rates in obstruction. (from Johnson RJ, Feehally J 2000 Comprehensive nephrology. Mosby Year Book.)

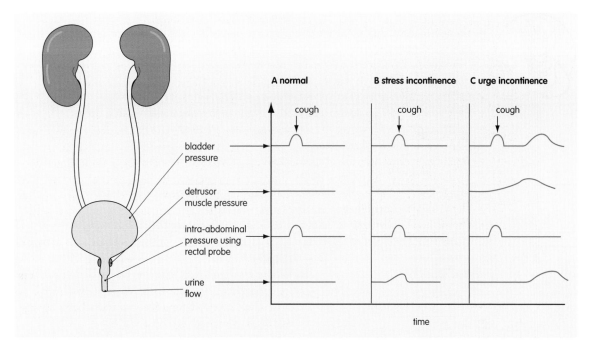

Fig. 8.20 Diagnosing incontinence using urodynamic studies. A, Normal cough; B, identifies stress incontinence, in which urine leakage is seen in response to a raised intra-abdominal pressure; C, shows urge incontinence, in which urine leakage is seen in response to detrusor muscle instability following a rise in intra-abdominal pressure.

Fig. 8.21 This bone scintigram shows areas of increased activity in the ribs, sternum and pelvis (highlighted on the scan as dark 'hotspolb'). This indicates multiple bone metastases in a patient with carcinoma of the prostate (courtesy Dr TO Nunan).

- Name five tests that can be performed on a urine sample, and explain the importance of an MSU sample.
- Describe the blood tests that can be done to investigate renal function, and give the possible causes of abnormal results.
- Give two reasons why plasma creatinine is a poor indicator of renal function.
- Explain when you would use ultrasonography in preference to plain radiography.
- List four contraindications and four complications of a renal biopsy.
- Explain how you would conduct an IVU.
- Describe the complications of specialist investigations involving the use of contrast medium.
- Explain the main differences between a diagnostic and therapeutic cystoscopy.
- Name the main investigation used to stage renal tumours.
- Explain how urodynamics studies can be used to differentiate between genuine stress incontinence and urge incontinence.

SELF-ASSESSMENT

Multiple-choice Questions (MCQs)

Indicate whether each answer is true or false.

1. Distribution of water:

(a) Intracellular fluid (ICF) accounts for one-third of total body water (TBW).
(b) The major cation of ICF is K^+.
(c) Extracellular fluid (ECF) is composed of interstitial fluid, plasma and transcellular fluid.
(d) The major anions of ECF are Cl^- and HCO_3^-.
(e) Inulin is used to measure ICF.

---

2. Potassium excretion by the kidney varies according to:

(a) The electric profile of the distal nephron (i.e. degree of electronegativity of tubule lumen compared with that of blood).
(b) Urine flow rate.
(c) Urinary Na^+ concentration.
(d) Urine pH.
(e) Plasma aldosterone concentration.

---

3. Subjects A and B are 70-kg males. Subject A drinks 2 L of distilled water and Subject B drinks 2 L of isotonic NaCl. As a result, subject B will have:

(a) Greater change in ICF volume.
(b) Higher positive free water clearance.
(c) Greater change in plasma osmolarity.
(d) Higher urine osmolarity.
(e) Higher urine flow rate.

---

4. The following can be measured directly:

(a) Total body water.
(b) Blood volume.
(c) Plasma volume.
(d) Intracellular volume.
(e) Interstitial fluid (ISF).

---

5. The following ions have a higher concentration in ECF than in ICF:

(a) Na^+.
(b) K^+.
(c) Cl^-.
(d) HCO_3^-.
(e) Ca^{2+}.

---

6. Regarding the loop of Henle:

(a) All nephrons have loops of Henle that enter the medulla.
(b) The thin descending loop is impermeable to water.
(c) The thin ascending loop is impermeable to water.
(d) The thick ascending loop transports sodium in the same way as the proximal tubule.
(e) ADH acts on the descending loop of Henle to increase its permeability to water.

---

7. A woman with a history of severe diarrhoea has the following arterial blood values: pH 7.25, pCO_2 3.2 kPa, HCO_3^- 10 mmol/L. The correct diagnosis is:

(a) Normal acid–base status.
(b) Metabolic acidosis.
(c) Metabolic alkalosis.
(d) Respiratory acidosis.
(e) Respiratory alkalosis.

---

8. Match the following blood gas results with one of the clinical situations listed below: pH 7.3, pCO_2 5.8 kPa, pO_2 8.0 kPa:

(a) Hyperventilation.
(b) Diabetic ketoacidosis.
(c) Pyloric stenosis.
(d) Morphine.
(e) High altitude.

---

9. Match the following blood gas results with one of the clinical situations listed below: pH 7.5, pCO_2 3.7 kPa, pO_2 14.4 kPa:

(a) Hyperventilation.
(b) Diabetic ketoacidosis.
(c) Pyloric stenosis.
(d) Mild asthma.
(e) COAD.

---

10. Match the following blood gas results with one of the clinical situations listed below: pH 7.34, pCO_2 7.3 kPa, pO_2 8.8 kPa:

(a) Hyperventilation.
(b) Diabetic ketoacidosis.
(c) Pyloric stenosis.
(d) Antacid ingestion.
(e) COAD.

11. Glomerular filtration rate is:

(a) Altered by eating a high protein meal.
(b) Accurately measured by *p*-aminohippuric acid (PAH) clearance.
(c) About 20% of plasma flow.
(d) Modified by the macula densa.
(e) About 180L per day.

12. The anion gap:

(a) Is normally 20–25 mmol/L.
(b) Is increased in renal tubular acidosis.
(c) Is normal after salicylate ingestion.
(d) Can be abnormal in chronic uraemia.
(e) Is affected by lactic acidosis.

13. Plasma creatinine concentration:

(a) Is never affected by diet.
(b) Is a sensitive guide to mild renal impairment.
(c) Depends upon weight.
(d) Is disproportionately increased compared with urea in rhabdomyolysis.
(e) Reflects glomerular filtration.

14. Which of the following would increase glomerular filtration rate (GFR)?

(a) Hyperproteinaemia.
(b) A ureteral stone.
(c) Dilatation of the afferent arteriole.
(d) Dilatation of the efferent arteriole.
(e) Constriction of the efferent arteriole.

15. Regarding plasma calcium levels:

(a) This is primarily regulated by the kidney.
(b) Hypercalcaemia is seen in rickets.
(c) Hypocalcaemia can cause constipation.
(d) Is inversely proportional to plasma phosphate concentration.
(e) Is always protein-bound in the blood.

16. Regarding plasma potassium levels:

(a) 98% of potassium is in the plasma.
(b) They can fall in patients taking steroids.
(c) Potassium disturbances can be asymptomatic.
(d) Potassium is actively reabsorbed in the proximal tubule.
(e) Potassium is lowered by aldosterone.

17. Regarding magnesium homeostasis:

(a) Plasma concentration is usually 2.12–2.60 mmol/L.
(b) It is important as it has a role in energy production.
(c) Magnesium is mainly protein bound in the plasma.
(d) Thiazide diuretics can cause hypomagnesaemia.
(e) Is mainly in the plasma.

18. Magnesium handling involves:

(a) Reabsorption, mainly in the proximal tubule.
(b) A cotransporter system in the loop of Henle.
(c) Intrinsic regulation by the cells of the thin descending loop of Henle.
(d) T_m limited absorption.
(e) Parathyroid hormone increases magnesium reabsorption in the thick ascending loop of Henle.

19. ADH:

(a) Is synthesized in the kidney.
(b) Acts on the collecting tubules.
(c) Has a plasma half-life of 5h.
(d) Release is triggered by hypernatraemia.
(e) Is mainly excreted in the urine.

20. High renin levels are associated with:

(a) Hyperaldosteronism.
(b) Addison's disease.
(c) Increased potassium intake.
(d) Captopril.
(e) Renal artery stenosis (RAS).

21. Which of the following would distinguish a healthy person with severe water deprivation from a person with syndrome of inappropriate antidiuretic hormone (SIADH)?

(a) Clearance of free water.
(b) Urine osmolarity.
(c) Plasma osmolarity.
(d) Circulating levels of ADH.
(e) Effective treatment with demeclocycline.

22. Acute renal failure (ARF):

(a) Can be caused by Wegener's granulomatosis.
(b) Can be irreversible.
(c) Is always associated with abnormalities on urine dipstick.
(d) Is a recognized complication of non-steroidal anti-inflammatory drug (NSAID) use.
(e) Can be treated effectively by dopamine infusion.

23. Nephrotic syndrome can be caused by:

(a) Gold.
(b) Penicillamine.
(c) Staphylococcal infection.
(d) Captopril.
(e) Paracetamol.

24. The following can be features of the nephritic syndrome:

(a) Oliguria.
(b) Low blood pressure.
(c) Haematuria.
(d) Decreased serum urea and creatinine.
(e) Evidence of a recent streptococcal infection.

25. Urinary tract obstruction:

(a) Is most often congenital in children.
(b) Is most common in men over 60 years of age.
(c) Is confined to the ureter.
(d) Can present as renal colic.
(e) Does not predispose to infection.

26. Diabetic nephropathy:

(a) Is more frequent in non-insulin-dependent diabetes mellitus (NIDDM) than insulin-dependent diabetes mellitus (IDDM).
(b) Is rare before 20 years of age.
(c) Can present as the nephrotic syndrome.
(d) Once present, usually progresses to end-stage renal failure.
(e) Is characterized by microhaematuria.

27. Adrenocortical insufficiency:

(a) Results in decreased osmolarity of ECF.
(b) Results in increased ECF volume.
(c) Results in increased haematocrit.
(d) Can occur after prolonged corticosteroid administration.
(e) Results in hypokalaemia.

28. Thiazide diuretics:

(a) Cause metabolic acidosis.
(b) Cause hyperuricaemia.
(c) Cause glucose intolerance.
(d) Cause hypocalcaemia.
(e) Are used in the treatment of angina.

29. The following statements are correct:

(a) The kidneys receive approximately 20% of the cardiac output.
(b) In healthy young adults approximately 120ml/min of protein-free filtrate is formed at the glomeruli.
(c) Non-protein-bound drugs of molecular weight less than 66kDa pass into the filtrate.
(d) Potentially saturable mechanisms for active secretion of both acids and bases exist in the proximal tubule.
(e) Low lipid solubility favours tubular reabsorption.

30. The following can impair renal function:

(a) Naproxen.
(b) Ranitidine.
(c) Iodine-containing contrast media.
(d) Captopril.
(e) Amphotericin B.

31. To maintain normal H^+ balance, total daily excretion of H^+ should equal the daily:

(a) Fixed acid production plus fixed acid ingestion.
(b) HCO_3^- excretion.
(c) HCO_3^- filtered load.
(d) Potassium excretion.
(e) Filtered load of H^+.

32. The following are secreted by the proximal tubule:

(a) Sodium.
(b) Potassium.
(c) Glucose.
(d) Bicarbonate.
(e) p-aminohippuric acid (PAH).

33. Production of urea is increased by:

(a) Old age.
(b) A low protein diet.
(c) Tetracycline.
(d) Glucocorticosteroid therapy.
(e) Surgery.

34. Renin release is controlled by:

(a) Osmotic concentration in the distal tubule.
(b) Pressure changes in the efferent arterioles.
(c) Parasympathetic tone.
(d) Local prostaglandin release.
(e) Angiotensin II.

35. Regarding resting renal blood flow:

(a) The glomerular filtration pressure is about 80mmHg.
(b) 10000 nephrons receive 1.2L of blood/min.
(c) The glomerular capillaries are supplied by the afferent arterioles.
(d) The afferent arterioles supply blood directly to the distal tubules.
(e) The blood supply of the medulla arises from the efferent arterioles.

36. Erythropoietin secretion can be increased by:

(a) ACE inhibitors.
(b) Hypoxia.
(c) Renal cell carcinoma.
(d) Loss of renal substance.
(e) Nephrotic syndrome.

37. Glomerulonephritis (GN):

(a) Affects both kidneys.
(b) Can be caused by immune complex disease.
(c) Is always the result of deposition of antiglomerular basement membrane (anti-GBM) antibody.
(d) Is always associated with pyelonephritis.
(e) Is associated with red cell casts on urine microscopy.

38. Life-threatening complications of acute glomerulonephritis include:

(a) Hypertensive encephalopathy.
(b) Pulmonary oedema.
(c) Uraemia.
(d) Epilepsy.
(e) Stroke.

39. The renal excretion of water is dependent upon:

(a) GFR.
(b) Reabsorption of solute in the proximal tubule.
(c) Concentration of ADH.
(d) Normal functioning distal convoluted tubule.
(e) Solute concentration in the thick ascending limb of the loop of Henle.

40. Factors that encourage the formation of urinary tract stones (urolithiasis) include:

(a) Cushing's syndrome.
(b) Dehydration.
(c) Hypocalcaemia.
(d) Urinary tract infection (UTI).
(e) Pregnancy.

41. Clinical features of urinary tract stones are:

(a) Asymptomatic.
(b) Haematuria.
(c) Renal colic.
(d) UTI.
(e) Urinary tract obstruction.

42. Regarding potassium metabolism:

(a) Intracellular potassium concentration is 150 mmol/L.
(b) Cellular uptake of potassium is decreased by insulin.
(c) Normal dietary intake is about 2–3 g/day.
(d) 20% of filtered potassium is excreted in the urine.
(e) Depletion of potassium is associated with metabolic alkalosis.

43. Predisposing factors in UTI are:

(a) Vesicoureteric reflux (VUR).
(b) Diabetes mellitus.
(c) Postmenopausal lack of oestrogen.
(d) Neurogenic bladder.
(e) Structural urinary tract abnormality.

44. Urinary tract infection (UTI):

(a) Is defined as over 10^7 organisms/mL in a midstream urine sample.
(b) Is more common in adult females.
(c) Is usually due to *Proteus* species organisms.
(d) Often occurs in children.
(e) Is usually attributed to infection from the patient's own faecal flora.

45. Recurrent urinary tract infection can be prevented by:

(a) Voiding before and after sexual intercourse.
(b) Voiding at regular 2–3-h intervals.
(c) Adequate control of diabetes.
(d) A 2 L daily intake of fluid.
(e) Immunosuppressant treatment.

46. Renal causes of oedema include:

(a) Acute glomerulonephritis.
(b) Nephrotic syndrome.
(c) Renal failure.
(d) Bladder transitional cell carcinoma.
(e) Cystitis.

47. Vesicoureteric reflux (VUR):

(a) Can be congenital.
(b) Is usually due to abnormal entry of the ureters into the bladder.
(c) Usually resolves by adulthood.
(d) Can lead to renal failure.
(e) Is diagnosed by cystoscopy.

48. VUR:

(a) May be associated with other genitourinary anomalies.
(b) Is always due to a developmental anomaly of the vesicoureteric junction.
(c) Can lead to reflux nephropathy.
(d) Is usually seen in middle-aged women.
(e) May require prophylactic antibiotic treatment.

49. Nephrotic syndrome patients:

(a) Can have frothy urine.
(b) Are more likely to have coexisting ischaemic heart disease.
(c) Are always children.
(d) Are always diagnosed by renal biopsy.
(e) Are usually treated with dialysis.

50. Minimal glomerular disease:

(a) Is most common in early childhood.
(b) Is characterized by podocyte changes seen under the light microscope.
(c) Is associated with nephrotic syndrome.
(d) Is treated with antibiotics.
(e) Has a better prognosis in adults.

51. Regarding Goodpasture's syndrome:

(a) Glomerular basement membrane autoantibodies develop.
(b) Patients present with 'crescentic' glomerulonephritis.
(c) Renal function gradually deteriorates, resulting in chronic renal failure.
(d) Is associated with lung haemorrhage.
(e) Requires supportive treatment only.

52. Transitional cell carcinoma (TCC):

(a) Is more common in females.
(b) Is more common in cigarette smokers.
(c) Usually affects the urethra.
(d) Is a benign tumour.
(e) Is diagnosed by urine cytology and cystoscopy.

53. Regarding prostate cancer:

(a) It develops as a result of benign prostatic hypertrophy.
(b) It is always associated with a raised prostate-specific antigen (PSA).
(c) A digital rectal examination reveals a hard and irregular prostate.
(d) The lesions are usually found in the posterior aspect of the lobe.
(e) It can be treated with testosterone.

54. Schistosomiasis:

(a) Is the most common blood fluke infection in the UK.
(b) Presents commonly with recurrent haematuria.
(c) Settles in the liver and the kidneys.
(d) Can lead to cystitis.
(e) Requires conservative treatment only.

55. Acute renal failure (ARF) can be caused by:

(a) Sepsis.
(b) Polycystic kidney disease.
(c) Renovascular disease.
(d) Diabetes mellitus.
(e) Myeloma.

56. Renal transplant:

(a) The transplanted kidney is placed in the same anatomical position as the original kidney.
(b) Has a poor success rate.
(c) Requires immunosuppressant therapy to prevent rejection.
(d) Recurrence of the original disease may occur.
(e) Is associated with an increased incidence of malignancy.

57. Proliferative GN:

(a) Can cause rapidly progressive renal failure.
(b) Is associated with basement membrane thickening.
(c) Occurs in Alport's syndrome.
(d) Is never due to systemic lupus erythematosus (SLE).
(e) Is the most common cause of childhood nephrotic syndrome.

58. Renal artery stenosis (RAS):

(a) Develops due to atherosclerosis.
(b) Can be bilateral.
(c) Reduces renin secretion.
(d) Can cause the kidneys to shrink.
(e) Can cause hypertension.

59. Hydronephrosis:

(a) Is always congenital.
(b) Can be caused by posterior urethral valves.
(c) Can be associated with hydroureters.
(d) Never resolves spontaneously.
(e) Is always bilateral.

60. Risk factors for pyelonephritis include:

(a) Being male and under 40 years of age.
(b) Pregnancy.
(c) Diabetes mellitus.
(d) Vesicoureteric reflux.
(e) Previous urinary tract surgery.

61. Wilm's tumour:

(a) Usually affects adults.
(b) Is usually unilateral.
(c) Is usually benign.
(d) Presents most commonly as a painless abdominal mass.
(e) Long-term survival is over 80%.

62. Potter's syndrome:

(a) Is unilateral renal agenesis.
(b) Involves pulmonary hypoplasia.
(c) Is associated with polyhydramnios.
(d) Is incompatible with life.
(e) Clinical features include low-set ears and an underdeveloped mandible.

63. Polyarteritis nodosa (PAN) characteristically:

(a) Is more common in females.
(b) Presents in old age.
(c) May present with constitutional symptoms such as fever and arthralgia.
(d) Affects medium-sized arteries.
(e) Is associated with aneurysms.

64. IgA nephropathy:

(a) Presents with UTI.
(b) Is most common in India.
(c) Is associated with mesangial proliferation.
(d) Is treated effectively by dialysis.
(e) Has a worse prognosis in patients with hypertension.

65. Membranous glomerulonephropathy:

(a) Is characterized by basement membrane thickening.
(b) Is more common in females.
(c) Has a similar pathology to Henoch–Schönlein purpura (HSP).
(d) Usually presents acutely.
(e) Is mainly treated with renal replacement therapy.

66. Membranoproliferative glomerulonephritis (GN):

(a) Is usually secondary to systemic diseases such as SLE.
(b) Often involves activation of the classical complement pathway.
(c) Is commonly seen in men over the age of 40.
(d) Can be asymptomatic.
(e) Can recur following transplant.

67. Henoch–Schönlein purpura (HSP):

(a) Is an immune-complex-mediated disorder.
(b) Exclusively affects the kidney.
(c) Is more common in females.
(d) Predisposes to renal carcinoma later in life.
(e) Has a poor prognosis.

68. Wegener's granulomatosis:

(a) Usually presents by the age of 20.
(b) Is a necrotizing vasculitis.
(c) Is an inherited disease.
(d) Characteristically presents with a purpuric skin rash on the extensor surfaces.
(e) Can be treated by cyclophosphamide.

69. Characteristic features of Alport's syndrome include:

(a) X-linked inheritance.
(b) Oedema.
(c) Microscopic haematuria.
(d) Cataracts.
(e) Deficiency of galactosidase A.

70. Regarding renal manifestations in multiple myeloma:

(a) Patients can develop acute renal failure.
(b) Bence-Jones proteins are excreted in the urine.
(c) Tubular obstruction can develop.
(d) Patients present with urinary tract infection.
(e) Hypercalcaemia is often seen.

71. In malignant hypertension:

(a) There is a rapid increase in blood pressure.
(b) Aetiology involves hyaline membrane changes.
(c) Patients have increased plasma levels of aldosterone.
(d) Patients might have papilloedema.
(e) Renal function usually remains intact.

72. Chronic analgesic abuse is a risk factor for:

(a) Acute tubulointerstitial pyelonephritis.
(b) Chronic tubulointerstitial nephritis.
(c) Transitional cell carcinoma.
(d) Glomerulonephritis.
(e) IgA nephropathy.

73. The following conditions can present with microscopic haematuria:

(a) Diabetes mellitus.
(b) Polyarteritis nodosa.
(c) Toxin-induced interstitial nephritis.
(d) Amyloidosis.
(e) Heavy exercise.

74. Treatment with corticosteroids is beneficial in patients with glomerulonephritis caused by:

(a) A streptococcal throat infection.
(b) Polyarteritis nodosa.
(c) SLE.
(d) Bacterial endocarditis.
(e) Wegener's granulomatosis.

75. Loop diuretics:

(a) Are weak diuretics.
(b) Reduce calcium excretion.
(c) Act in the thin descending loop of Henle.
(d) Relieve pulmonary oedema.
(e) Can cause gynaecomastia.

76. ACE inhibitors:

(a) Inhibit the conversion of renin to angiotensin II.
(b) Relieve symptoms, and thus prolong life in congestive cardiac failure.
(c) Are safe in pregnancy.
(d) Can cause hyperkalaemia.
(e) Reduce proteinuria in diabetic nephropathy.

77. Regarding the anatomy of the lower urinary tract:

(a) The ureters are fully retroperitoneal.
(b) Ureteric obstruction can cause pain in the scrotum or labium majus.
(c) The bladder has a maximum capacity of 200 mL.
(d) The bladder neck moves freely as the bladder fills.
(e) The prostate gland is composed only of glandular tissue.

78. The following are risk factors for urinary tract stone formation:

(a) Hypercalcaemia.
(b) Hypercalciuria.
(c) Dehydration.
(d) Hypouricaemia.
(e) High spinach intake.

79. Causes of urinary tract obstruction include:

(a) Urethral strictures.
(b) Hydronephrosis.
(c) Prostate cancer.
(d) Urinary tract calculi.
(e) Pregnancy.

80. Urinary tract obstruction can present with:

(a) Renal colic.
(b) Hydronephrosis.
(c) Polyuria.
(d) Anuria.
(e) Stress incontinence.

81. Causes of acute tubular necrosis (ATN) include:

(a) Severe burns.
(b) Gentamicin.
(c) Vitamin A.
(d) Gold salts.
(e) Paracetamol overdose.

82. ATN:

(a) Can present initially with oliguria.
(b) Is reversible with supportive treatment.
(c) Is associated with hypokalaemia.
(d) Is never associated with sepsis.
(e) Is associated with small kidneys.

83. Management of chronic renal failure includes:

(a) A high protein diet.
(b) Regular checks on parathyroid hormones.
(c) Antihypertensive treatment.
(d) Correction of anaemia with erythropoietin.
(e) Renal replacement therapy.

84. The following are causes of metabolic acidosis:

(a) Vomiting.
(b) Insulin-dependent diabetes mellitus.
(c) Chronic renal failure.
(d) Salicylate poisoning.
(e) Hyperaldosteronism.

85. The following cause hyperkalaemia:

(a) Hyperaldosteronism.
(b) Alkalosis.
(c) Treatment with β-agonists (e.g. salbutamol).
(d) Insulin administration.
(e) Decreased serum osmolarity.

86. The right kidney:

(a) Lies posterior to the second part of the duodenum.
(b) Lies immediately lateral to the aorta.
(c) Is higher than the left kidney.
(d) Lies anterior to psoas muscle.
(e) Has a colonic impression on its anterior surface.

87. Benign prostatic hypertrophy (BPH):

(a) Occurs most often in men under 60 years of age.
(b) Is associated with median lobe enlargement.
(c) Acute retention requires surgical treatment.
(d) Can metastasize.
(e) Can present with UTI.

88. Renal cell carcinoma:

(a) Is the most common renal tumour in adults.
(b) Can present with bony metastases.
(c) Is associated with a high α-fetoprotein.
(d) Arises from the proximal tubule epithelium.
(e) Has an increased incidence in von Hippel–Lindau disease.

89. In adult polycystic disease of the kidney:

(a) The inheritance is autosomal dominant.
(b) Massive proteinuria is always found.
(c) The diagnosis is compatible with a normal life span.
(d) The cysts involve all parts of the nephron.
(e) There is a recognized association with intracerebral aneurysms.

90. Bladder transitional cell carcinoma (TCC):

(a) Is usually benign.
(b) Is associated with cigarette smoking.
(c) Has a higher incidence in Egypt.
(d) Presents with a painful haematuria.
(e) Usually occurs on the posterior and lateral walls of the bladder.

91. Causes of urge incontinence include:

(a) Congenital lesions.
(b) Multiple childbirth.
(c) Faecal impaction.
(d) Brain tumour.
(e) Alzheimer's disease.

92. Regarding stress incontinence:

(a) This is involuntary urine loss associated with an increase in intra-abdominal pressure.
(b) Is more common in females than in males.
(c) Usually develops in old age.
(d) Can be caused by urinary tract instrumentation.
(e) Is exacerbated by obesity.

93. Osmoreceptors:

(a) Detect variations in plasma osmolality.
(b) Are located in the thalamus.
(c) Receive blood supply from the internal carotid artery.
(d) Have no effect on thirst.
(e) Regulate the release of ADH.

94. ADH release is increased by:

(a) Nicotine.
(b) Angiotensin.
(c) Alcohol.
(d) Carbemazepine.
(e) β-blockers.

95. Unilateral kidney enlargement can be found in:

(a) Tumour.
(b) Benign cyst.
(c) Pyelonephritis.
(d) Hydronephrosis.
(e) Chronic renal failure.

96. An enlarged kidney:

(a) May be confused with an enlarged spleen.
(b) The superior surface can be palpated.
(c) Has a notched edge.
(d) Is more easily felt in children.
(e) Is usually painful.

97. Regarding urinary casts:

(a) Hyaline casts in urine are always pathological.
(b) The presence of up to five red blood cell casts in urine is normal.
(c) White cell casts are detected in acute pyelonephritis.
(d) Tubular cell casts are seen in acute tubular necrosis.
(e) Red cell casts are seen in nephrotic syndrome.

98. Ultrasound is useful to investigate renal disease because it can:

(a) Differentiate between solid and cystic masses.
(b) Provide infromation about the functional capacity of each kidney.
(c) Highlight the anatomy of the ureters.
(d) Identify prostatic enlargement in males.
(e) Provide evidence of rejection in a transplanted kidney.

99. Renal biopsy:

(a) Is used to classify glomerulonephritis histologically.
(b) Is performed frequently in children.
(c) Requires ultrasound guidance.
(d) Can lead to a perinephric haematoma.
(e) Is contraindicated if the kidneys are small.

100. Regarding renal imaging:

(a) A 'kidney/ureter/bladder' (KUB) X-ray is the same as an abdominal X-ray.
(b) Plain radiography always detects calculi.
(c) A micturating cystogram is used to confirm vesicoureteric reflux.
(d) Computed tomography (CT) is used to stage renal tumours.
(e) Renal arteriography involves contrast injected into the renal vein.

Short-answer Questions (SAQs)

1. Outline the functions of the kidneys.

2. Describe the renal blood supply.

3. Write short notes on the fetal development of the urinary system.

4. Give two examples of how failure of the normal development of renal tract can lead to anatomical abnormalities.

5. Write short notes on the structure of the glomerular filter.

6. Write short notes on the transport processes of the renal tubule.

7. How are the glomerular filtration rate (GFR) and renal blood flow (RBF) measured?

8. Summarize the age-related changes in RBF and GFR?

9. Discuss the transport of glucose in the proximal tubule and how this correlates with plasma glucose levels.

10. Discuss the reabsorption of bicarbonate ions in the proximal tubule.

11. Draw the adult nephron and label the afferent and efferent arterioles, glomerulus and tubular segments.

12. Summarize the effects of diabetes on the kidney.

13. Outline the mechanism used by angiotensin-converting enzyme (ACE) inhibitors to reduce hypertension.

14. Write short notes on renal artery stenosis (RAS) and explain why ACE inhibitors are contraindicated in patients with RAS.

15. Summarize the five main mechanisms of glomerular injury, illustrating each with a clinical example.

16. Write short notes on the complications of benign prostatic hypertrophy.

17. A 62-year-old known hypertensive presents with a left-sided stroke. Examination reveals a blood pressure of 173/100mmHg, with xanthelasma and xanthoma. Bilateral corneal arcus is seen and bilateral abdominal bruits and a right-sided carotid bruit can be heard. Urine electrolytes revealed an elevated plasma creatinine of 240µmol/L. Blood cholesterol is elevated.
    (a) What is the significance of the bruits?
    (b) What is the diagnosis?
    (c) Which investigation would confirm this?
    (d) Why are ACE inhibitors contraindicated in this patient?
    (e) Does the patient require dialysis?
    (f) Name three aspects of management.

18. A 74-year-old man presents with difficulty in starting micturition and a poor urinary stream with dribbling at the end of the stream. He also has nocturia, waking up six times a night to pass urine.
    (a) What must be included in the clinical examination?
    (b) What are the main differentials?
    (c) What blood test can be performed to confirm the diagnosis?

19. A 7-year-old Asian boy presents with a 3-day history of oedema around the eyes, which is worse on waking. The parents report a reduced urine output, which appears 'frothy'. Examination reveals ankle and abdominal oedema, with reduced breath sounds (particularly on the right). There is also some scrotal swelling.
    (a) What is the most likely diagnosis?
    (b) List three useful investigations.
    (c) Describe the management of this child.

20. A 35-year-old man presents with painful micturition. In particular, he finds the pain worse at the end of micturition, sometimes spreading to his penis. The pain is exacerbated by sudden movements, and is relieved by lying down. Over the last week, he has also noticed that the urine appears bloody towards the end of micturition.
    (a) What is the most likely cause of the pain?
    (b) Why is the pain referred to the penis, and why is it relieved on lying down?
    (c) What is the investigation of choice to confirm the suspected diagnosis?

Essay Questions

1. Describe the methods used to measure body fluid compartments including: (a) plasma volume, red cell volume and blood volume, (b) extracellular fluid (ECF), (c) interstitial fluid (ISF), (d) total body water (TBW), (e) transcellular fluid (TCF).

2. Discuss the various anatomical sections of the loop of Henle and how this acts as a countercurrent multiplier.

3. Give an account of the actions and side-effects of the five classes of diuretics.

4. Compare and contrast acute and chronic renal failure.

5. Discuss the conditions associated with abnormal or inappropriate ADH secretion.

6. Outline the renin–angiotensin–aldosterone system, highlighting its clinical significance. Summarize the drugs that alter this system.

7. Discuss the renal handling of sodium, explaining how this can vary under different circumstances.

8. Discuss the predisposition, presentation and complications of urinary tract infections.

9. Compare and contrast the reabsorption of salts and water in the proximal convoluted tubule with that in the distal convoluted tubule and cortical collecting duct.

10. Discuss the role of the kidney in regulation of acid–base balance.

11. Give an account of potassium regulation in the kidney, considering the clinical features and causes of disturbances and the consequences if untreated.

12. Discuss the possible congenital abnormalities of the kidney and urinary tract, and their clinical significance.

13. Give an account of the causes, possible presentations and management of both unilateral and bilateral urinary tract obstruction.

14. Discuss the common presentations of renal disease, and the possible underlying causes.

15. Outline the systemic disorders that can cause glomerular disease, clarifying the main histological abnormalities.

16. Discuss the possible carcinomas seen in: (a) the kidney, (b) the bladder.

17. Compare and contrast the methods involved in renal replacement therapy.

18. Discuss the management of a patient presenting with haematuria.

19. Give an account of the various types of renal imaging, explaining the indications and limitations for each.

20. Discuss the diseases of the renal blood vessels.

MCQ Answers

1. (a) F—ICF accounts for two-thirds TBW.
    (b) T—The major ECF cation is sodium.
    (c) T—Together, this accounts for one-third of TBW.
    (d) T—These are both found in low concentrations in intracellular fluid.
    (e) F—Inulin is used to estimate GFR.

2. (a) T—Renal tubule acidosis can cause hypokalaemia in the distal tubule.
    (b) T—Flow rate in the collecting duct decreases lumen potassium, and thus increases potassium secretion.
    (c) T—This is inversely proportional to potassium excretion.
    (d) T—Potassium is excreted in association with H^+, so its excretion increases with a low blood pH.
    (e) T—This increases potassium excretion.

3. (a) F—Distilled water is a hypotonic solution, which draws water out of cells.
    (b) F—Water accompanies NaCl excretion in subject B; subject A has no extra NaCl, so free water clearance is higher.
    (c) F—Isotonic solutions have the same concentration as plasma.
    (d) T—Subject B excretes extra NaCl, which increases urine osmolarity.
    (e) F—This is not altered.

4. (a) T—This is measured using isotopes of water as markers.
    (b) F—This is a combination of plasma and erythrocyte volume.
    (c) T—This can be measured using radiolabelled albumin.
    (d) F—This is the difference between total body water and extracellular fluid.
    (e) F—ISF = extracellular fluid – plasma volume.

5. (a) T—This is the main extracellular cation.
    (b) F—This is the main intracellular cation.
    (c) T—ECF [Cl^-] = 113 mmol/L; ICF [Cl^-] = 4 mmol/L.
    (d) T—ECF [HCO_3^-] = 27 mmol/L; ICF [HCO_3^-] = 12 mmol/L.
    (e) T—50% of total body calcium is found in the ECF.

6. (a) F—Only 15% of nephrons extend into the medulla.
    (b) F—It is water permeable.
    (c) T—It is water impermeable.
    (d) F—The cotransporters are different.
    (e) F—ADH acts on the collecting duct.

7. (a) F—Normal blood pH is 7.35–7.45.
    (b) T—HCO_3^- is reduced, so pH falls.
    (c) F—Blood pH increases in alkalosis.
    (d) F—Diarrhoea does not affect the respiratory system, and pCO_2 is normal.
    (e) F—Blood pH increases in alkalosis.

8. (a) F—This causes alkalosis and an increase in blood pH.
    (b) F—This causes a metabolic acidosis, with no change in pCO_2 and pO_2.
    (c) F—This leads to vomiting, which causes a metabolic alkalosis.
    (d) T—This acts as a respiratory centre depressant.
    (e) F—This is associated with a respiratory alkalosis.

9. (a) T—Overbreathing increases CO_2 loss, which causes a respiratory alkalosis (pH increases).
    (b) F—This is associated with a metabolic acidosis.
    (c) F—This is alkalosis primarily due to metabolic causes.
    (d) F—This causes a respiratory acidosis.
    (e) F—As (d).

10. (a) F—This has a low pCO_2 and an elevated pH.
    (b) F—pH falls in diabetic ketoacidosis, resulting in a metabolic acidosis.
    (c) F—This does not reduce pO_2.
    (d) F—Ingestion of alkali causes a metabolic alkalosis.
    (e) T—This is associated with a gradual increase in pCO_2 and consequently there is a fall in pH.

11. (a) T—Protein metabolism produces H^+ ions; excess acid must be excreted in urine to prevent acidosis.
    (b) F—This measures renal plasma flow.
    (c) T—GFR = 120 mL/min.
    (d) T—This detects changes in the pressure/flow within the kidney.
    (e) T—GFR is 120 mL/min, which is 180 L per day (both kidneys).

12. (a) F—It is usually between 8 and 16 mmol/L.
    (b) F—The difference between plasma anions and cations is unchanged.
    (c) F—This increases the anion gap.
    (d) T—Chronic uraemia leads to acidosis, which causes an increased anion gap.
    (e) T—Excess metabolic production of acid increases the anion gap.

13. (a) F—Creatinine is produced in muscle, and is higher in people with larger muscle bulk.
    (b) F—Creatinine clearance overestimates the GFR, because there is tubular creatinine secretion.
    (c) T—Muscle bulk influences creatinine levels.
    (d) T—This is muscle breakdown, resulting in creatinine release.
    (e) T—Creatinine clearance is used to estimate GFR.

14. (a) F—High blood protein levels do not alter the rate of filtration.
    (b) F—This affects urine flow, not filtration rate.
    (c) T—This increases renal perfusion pressure.
    (d) F—This does not alter the rate at which blood is filtered, it alters the rate of blood flow.
    (e) T—This restricts the maximum rate at which blood can flow out of the glomerulus.

15. (a) T—This is the main site of calcium reabsorption or excretion.
    (b) F—Rickets is due to hypocalcaemia with a low vitamin D.
    (c) F—Hypercalcaemia causes a fall in intestinal motility, thus causing constipation.
    (d) T—A rise in plasma calcium leads to a fall in plasma phosphate.
    (e) F—Ionized calcium is also seen.

16. (a) F—98% is in the intracellular fluid.
    (b) T—Corticosteroids increase potassium excretion.
    (c) T—Symptoms develop as the severity of the potassium deficit increases.
    (d) F—80–90% of potassium is passively reabsorbed in the proximal tubule.
    (e) T—Aldosterone stimulates potassium secretion and thus its excretion.

17. (a) T—Plasma magnesium levels are under strict control.
    (b) T—Magnesium controls mitochondrial oxidate metabolism.
    (c) F—20% of magnesium is protein bound.
    (d) T—Thiazide diuretics increase magnesium excretion together with potassium loss.
    (e) F—Over 90% of magnesium is found in the bone and in cells.

18. (a) F—Only 15% of magnesium is reabsorbed in the proximal tubule.
    (b) T—This is present in the thick ascending loop.
    (c) F—Regulation is by the thick ascending loop of Henle.
    (d) T—If T_m is exceeded, magnesium is excreted in the urine.
    (e) T—PTH also increases calcium reabsorption.

19. (a) F—It is synthesized in the hypothalamus.
    (b) T—This is the main site of action.
    (c) F—Plasma half-life is 10–15 min.
    (d) T—ADH is secreted in response to increased plasma osmolality.
    (e) F—Less than 10% appears in the urine.

20. (a) F—This lowers renin levels by negative feedback.
    (b) T—Low plasma sodium stimulates renin secretion.
    (c) F—Renin secretion is influenced by sodium levels, not potassium levels.
    (d) T—Captopril is an ACE inhibitor, so no aldosterone is released and there is no negative feedback to inhibit renin release.
    (e) T—Renin is released because there is renal hypoperfusion in RAS.

21. (a) F—This can be normal.
    (b) F—A concentrated urine is typical in SIADH, but can also be seen in a healthy person.
    (c) T—SIADH patients have a low plasma osmolarity.
    (d) F—Plasma ADH levels vary in a healthy person.
    (e) T—This opposes ADH actions, and is used in patients with hyponatraemia due to excessive ADH secretion.

22. (a) T—This is a systemic vasculitis with renal manifestations.
    (b) T—If ARF is due to ischaemic necrosis, this is irreversible unless detected early.
    (c) F—Dipstix may not detect changes seen in ATN, the commonest cause of ARF.
    (d) T—NSAIDs cause minimal change glomerular disease, with nephrotic syndrome.
    (e) F—This is used to promote renal blood flow; it does not have a role in ARF.

23. (a) T—This causes a membranous nephropathy, which leads to nephrotic syndrome.
    (b) T—This also causes a membranous nephropathy.
    (c) F—This does not cause proteinuria.
    (d) T—This is an ACE inhibitor, which causes proteinuria if taken in large doses.
    (e) F—This does not impair glomerular filtration.

24. (a) T—Acute renal impairment is usually associated with a fall in urine production.
    (b) F—Renal impairment in nephritic syndrome is usually associated with a fall in urine output, and thus blood pressure increases.
    (c) T—This is due to glomerular injury.
    (d) F—Serum urea and creatinine may be normal or elevated.
    (e) T—This is post-streptococcal glomerular nephritis.

25. (a) T—It is usually due to structural abnormalities.
    (b) T—This is related to prostate enlargement.
    (c) F—Obstruction can occur in the urethra or the renal pelvis.
    (d) T—Smooth muscle contracts to expel the obstruction, resulting in colicky pain.
    (e) F—Obstruction impedes urine flow, causing stasis and thus predisposing to infection.

26. (a) F—IDDM has a younger onset, so patients have long-standing diabetes, which predisposes to nephropathy.
    (b) T—Nephropathy is a complication of long-standing, poorly controlled diabetes.
    (c) T—Severe proteinuria causes nephrotic syndrome.
    (d) T—Diabetes is the most common cause of end-stage renal disease.
    (e) F—It is characterized by microalbuminaemia in the early stages.

27. (a) T—No aldosterone is secreted, so sodium reabsorption is limited.
    (b) F—Sodium and water is lost, so the ECF volume is depleted.
    (c) T—There is volume depletion without a fall in the number of red blood cells, so the haematocrit increases.
    (d) T—The adrenocortex adjusts to exogenous corticosteroid therapy, so there is a deficiency once these are stopped.
    (e) F—A decrease in aldosterone reduces potassium excretion.

28. (a) F—Diuretics cause hypokalaemia, which is life-threatening.
    (b) T—Cholesterol levels can also rise.
    (c) T—Hyperglycaemia can result.
    (d) F—Calcium reabsorption is increased.
    (e) F—They are used to treat hypertension and congestive cardiac failure.

29. (a) T—The kidneys receive 1.2L/min of blood.
    (b) T—This is the GFR.
    (c) T—Substances over 70kDa are too large to pass into the filtrate.
    (d) T—This is driven by a sodium gradient, so sodium is reabsorbed simultaneously.
    (e) F—Lipid-soluble substances can be reabsorbed.

30. (a) T—This is a non-steroidal drug, which can cause minimal change glomerular disease.
    (b) F—This does not affect renal function.
    (c) T—An acute allergic reaction to the contrast can lead to renal failure.
    (d) T—This is an ACE inhibitor, which reduces aldosterone secretion, thus causing polyuria.
    (e) T—This is an antifungal drug, which can cause toxin-induced interstitial nephritis.

31. (a) T—This alters daily.
    (b) F—H^+ excretion is influenced by HCO_3^-, but does not equal it.
    (c) F—This does not influence H^+ excretion.
    (d) F—This is lost in association with H^+.
    (e) F—Some of the filtered H^+ must be reabsorbed.

32. (a) F—65% of filtered sodium is reabsorbed in the proximal tubule.
    (b) F—Potassium is not secreted by the kidney.
    (c) F—This is reabsorbed in the proximal tubule.
    (d) F—This is reabsorbed in the proximal tubule.
    (e) T—This is secreted in the pars recta.

33. (a) F—Protein breakdown does not increase with age.
    (b) F—Urea is produced from protein breakdown.
    (c) T—High doses reduce protein synthesis, resulting in increased amounts of unused urea.
    (d) T—Glucocorticosteroids increase protein catabolism, thereby increasing urea production.
    (e) T—Surgery stimulates protein breakdown, resulting in urea production.

34. (a) T—Renin release is stimulated by a fall in sodium in the distal tubule.
    (b) F—Renin is secreted in response to renal perfusion pressure, not efferent arteriolar pressure changes.
    (c) F—Sympathetic tone stimulates renin release.
    (d) T—Prostaglandins stimulate renin secretion directly.
    (e) T—Angiotensin II causes feedback inhibition of renin release.

35. (a) F—This is usually 90–200mmHg.
    (b) F—Together, both kidneys receive 1000mL/min.
    (c) T—These are sub-branches originating from the renal arteries.
    (d) F—The distal tubules are supplied by the efferent arterioles.
    (e) T—The medulla is supplied by the vasa recta from the efferent arterioles.

36. (a) F—ACE inhibitors reduce erythropoietin levels.
    (b) T—The mechanism for this is unclear.
    (c) T—The tumour cells can produce erythropoietin.
    (d) F—There are fewer cells available to secrete erythropoietin.
    (e) F—This involves faulty filtration, with no change in erythropoietin secretion.

37. (a) T—GN is usually immune mediated, and therefore blood borne.
    (b) T—An example is anti-DNA antibodies, as seen in SLE.
    (c) F—There are four other mechanisms resulting in GN.
    (d) F—Pyelonephritis is a bacterial infection of the kidney, GN is localized glomerular disease.
    (e) T—Haematuria is a feature of glomerular disease.

181

38. (a) T—Hypertension develops due to increased circulating fluid volume (because of oliguria/anuria).
    (b) T—This is due to fluid retention.
    (c) T—Glomerular filtering fails, so blood urate levels rise.
    (d) F—This is unrelated to acute GN.
    (e) F—This is linked to hypertension, not directly to GN.

39. (a) T—If GFR is low, less blood is filtered and less water is excreted.
    (b) T—Water is reabsorbed passively, following solute reabsorption.
    (c) T—ADH stimulates sodium and consequently water retention.
    (d) T—Principal cells in the distal tubules respond to ADH.
    (e) T—This creates a concentration gradient, which draws water back into the blood capillaries.

40. (a) T—Excess glucocorticoids predispose stone formation.
    (b) T—This increases the risk of infection, which predisposes stone formation.
    (c) F—Hypercalcaemia do associated with stone formation.
    (d) T—Infection increases the risk of solute deposition, and thus stone formation.
    (e) F—This is associated with incontinence, not stone formation.

41. (a) T—Stones can be detected incidentally.
    (b) T—This can be microscopic or macroscopic.
    (c) T—Pain occurs as the urinary tract muscle contracts to expel the stone.
    (d) T—Stones encourage organisms to harbour in the urinary tract.
    (e) T—As the stone enlarges, it can cause an obstruction.

42. (a) T—This is the main intracellular cation.
    (b) F—Insulin stimulates potassium uptake by cells.
    (c) T—Potassium is essential as it influences tissue excitability.
    (d) F—Only 5–15% of filtered potassium is excreted to maintain potassium balance.
    (e) T—Metabolic alkalosis is associated with a high pH and low H^+, which is associated with low K^+.

43. (a) T—Abnormal ureteric entry into the bladder causes reflux during voiding.
    (b) T—Excess glucose encourages bacterial growth.
    (c) T—Oestrogen stimulates vaginal secretions, which are bactericidal.
    (d) T—There is chronic urinary retention, which is at risk of infection.
    (e) T—An example is congenital ureteric strictures or abnormal ureteric bladder entry.

44. (a) F—This is defined as 10^5 organism/mL in a urine sample.
    (b) T—This is because the female urethra is shorter.
    (c) F—70% of UTIs are due to *E. coli*.
    (d) F—Any UTI in children must be investigated.
    (e) T—This often contaminates the urinary tract, leading to UTI.

45. (a) T—Intercourse introduces bacteria so flushing them out afterwards helps to prevent UTI.
    (b) T—This removes pathogens, preventing their accumulation in the urinary tract.
    (c) T—Glycosuria encourages bacterial growth in the urine.
    (d) T—A high fluid intake prevents a concentrated urine, thus reducing the risk of infection.
    (e) F—Immunosuppressants predispose to urinary tract infections.

46. (a) T—Oedema is seen due to a fall in urine output.
    (b) T—Oedema develops due to hypoproteinaemia.
    (c) T—Oedema occurs due to fluid retention.
    (d) F—This does not impede urine production.
    (e) F—This is bladder infection, which does not affect urine output.

47. (a) T—VUR can be congenital or acquired.
    (b) T—This is usually congenital.
    (c) T—Most of the damage is done by the age of five.
    (d) T—This is the result of chronic pyelonephritis and scarring.
    (e) F—Micturating cystourethrogram is used to show urine flow up the ureters while voiding.

48. (a) T—It can be associated with ureteric strictures.
    (b) F—It can be secondary to bladder pathology.
    (c) T—This is glomerular disease caused by backflow of urine into the kidney.
    (d) F—It is mostly seen in young boys (congenital), or patients with pre-existing bladder pathology.
    (e) T—Antibiotics are required to prevent infection and thus nephropathy.

49. (a) T—This is due to proteinuria.
    (b) T—This is due to hyperlipidaemia.
    (c) F—It can also present in adults.
    (d) F—Renal biopsy is not performed routinely in children.
    (e) F—Treatment is usually with glucocorticoids and supportive treatment (diuretics and ACE inhibitors).

50. (a) T—This is more common in children.
    (b) F—Podocyte fusion is seen only under the electron microscope.
    (c) T—This is the most common cause of nephrotic syndrome.
    (d) F—Treatment involves corticosteroids.
    (e) F—Prognosis is better in children.

51. (a) T—This is characteristic of Goodpasture's syndrome.
    (b) T—This can lead to acute renal failure.
    (c) F—Patients develop acute renal failure.
    (d) T—This is more common in smokers.
    (e) F—Patients require plasmaphoresis.

52. (a) F—The male:female ratio is 4:1.
    (b) T—Smoking is a risk factor for developing TCC.
    (c) F—Most TCCs arise in the bladder.
    (d) F—This is a malignant tumour.
    (e) T—Cystoscopy allows a clear view of the internal aspect of the bladder.

53. (a) F—This is a separate disorder.
    (b) F—A normal PSA does not exclude prostate cancer.
    (c) T—BPH is associated with a smooth enlarged prostate.
    (d) T—BPH lesions are usually more medial.
    (e) F—Testosterone stimulates tumour growth.

54. (a) F—This is rare in the UK, but is the most common fluke infection worldwide.
    (b) T—This is the most common presentation.
    (c) F—The pathogen settles in the bladder to lay eggs.
    (d) T—Schistosomiasis infection predisposes to cystitis.
    (e) F—Treatment involves praziquantel, given daily.

55. (a) T—This results in septicaemia, leading to ATN.
    (b) F—PKD is a cause of chronic renal failure, not ARF.
    (c) F—This can lead to CRF because of renal hypoperfusion and ischaemia.
    (d) F—Diabetes is a cause of chronic renal failure.
    (e) T—Myeloma can present with ARF.

56. (a) F—The transplanted kidney is placed in the iliac fossa.
    (b) F—Renal transplantation is one of the most successful organ transplants.
    (c) T—This is continued indefinitely.
    (d) T—This depends on the original aetiology of the disease.
    (e) T—It is associated with lymphomas in particular.

57. (a) T—Prognosis is therefore poor without treatment.
    (b) T—This is due to C3 deposition and mesangial proliferation.
    (c) F—This results in a mutation in glomerular basement membrane collagen.
    (d) F—A diffuse or focal proliferative GN is seen in SLE.
    (e) F—Minimal change nephropathy accounts for 90% of nephrotic syndrome seen in children.

58. (a) T—Atheromatous plaques deposit within the renal wall.
    (b) T—Bilateral abdominal bruits may be heard.
    (c) F—Renin secretion increases due to renal hypoperfusion.
    (d) T—This is a long-term change.
    (e) T—RAS stimulates renin and therefore aldosterone release, which promotes salt and water retention.

59. (a) F—It can develop as a result of stenosis.
    (b) T—These impede urine flow down the urinary tract.
    (c) T—The ureters gradually dilate to accommodate extra fluid.
    (d) F—Mild hydronephrosis can resolve spontaneously.
    (e) F—It is unilateral if due to obstruction and bilateral if due to posterior urethral valves.

60. (a) F—Women are more at risk between puberty and their late 50s.
    (b) T—Smooth muscle relaxation leads to reflux.
    (c) T—Glucose in the urine encourages bacterial growth.
    (d) T—Urine reflux exposes the kidney to infection.
    (e) T—Postoperative infection can develop.

61. (a) F—This usually presents in children under 10 years old.
    (b) T—Approximately 5% are bilateral.
    (c) F—Lung metastases are common.
    (d) T—Haematuria, pain or fever are also common.
    (e) T—Treatment involves nephrectomy and chemotherapy.

62. (a) F—It is bilateral renal agenesis.
    (b) T—This presents with respiratory distress at birth.
    (c) F—Potter's syndrome is associated with oligohydramnios.
    (d) T—The baby might be stillborn.
    (e) T—These are characteristic features.

63. (a) F—This has equal sex incidence.
    (b) T—It is commonly associated with giant cell arteritis.
    (c) T—This is a systemic disorder.
    (d) T—In comparison, microscopic PAN affects the small arteries of the body.
    (e) T—PAN is a necrotizing vasculitis.

64. (a) F—It usually presents with haematuria or proteinuria.
    (b) F—It is most common in France, Australia and Singapore.
    (c) T—C3 and IgA is also deposited in the mesangium.
    (d) F—There is no effective treatment.
    (e) T—Hypertension is associated with raised IgA levels.

65. (a) T—There is also subepithelial deposition of immune complexes.
    (b) F—It is more common in males.
    (c) T—A membranous nephropathy might be seen in HSP.
    (d) F—This is a chronic disease, with gradual onset.
    (e) F—Drug treatments include corticosteroids, ciclosporin and cyclophosphamide.

66. (a) F—This is usually a primary GN.
    (b) F—It involves the alternate complement pathway.
    (c) F—This is seen mainly in children and young adults.
    (d) T—It can also present with haematuria or nephrotic/nephritic syndrome.
    (e) T—This depends on the original cause of the GN.

67. (a) F—It is a vasculitis.
    (b) F—It also affects the skin, joints and the gut.
    (c) F—It is more common in males under the age of 10.
    (d) F—There is no association with a carcinoma.
    (e) F—Prognosis is good.

68. (a) F—It most commonly affects 40–50-year-olds.
    (b) T—It usually affects the kidneys, nose and upper respiratory tract.
    (c) F—It is not inherited.
    (d) F—This is characteristic of HSP.
    (e) T—Treatment must be started as early as possible.

69. (a) T—There might also be autosomal dominant or recessive inheritance.
    (b) F—Presentation is with haematuria or GN.
    (c) T—This is due to an abnormal basement membrane structure.
    (d) T—Ocular lesions are common.
    (e) F—This is seen in Fabry's syndrome.

70. (a) T—This is because of acute renal insufficiency.
    (b) T—Excess antibodies saturate the reabsorption mechanism, spilling into the urine.
    (c) T—This is because of cast deposition.
    (d) F—Asymptomatic renal failure is commonly found.
    (e) T—This is because of bone erosion.

71. (a) T—It is associated with malignant hypertension.
    (b) F—This is seen in essential hypertension.
    (c) T—This is because of a rise in renin secretion.
    (d) T—This is a manifestation of hypertension.
    (e) F—Patients can develop renal failure.

72. (a) T—This can occur as a result of long-standing tubular inflammation.
    (b) T—T-cell-mediated inflammation causes chronic nephritis.
    (c) T—Analgesic abuse is a risk factor for TCC.
    (d) F—Analgesic abuse does not affect the glomerulus in isolation.
    (e) F—This is because of IgA deposition in the glomeruli, which is not associated with analgesic abuse.

73. (a) F—This can present with proteinuria.
    (b) T—Haematuria occurs because this is a necrotizing vasculitis, leaking blood into the urine.
    (c) T—Haematuria results from T-cell-mediated inflammation.
    (d) F—This usually presents with proteinuria or nephrotic syndrome.
    (e) F—This can result in haemoglobinuria.

74. (a) F—This requires antibiotic treatment.
    (b) T—This is a systemic vasculitis, effectively treated with steroids.
    (c) T—This is a connective tissue disorder, which requires steroid treatment.
    (d) F—This requires prophylactic antibiotics.
    (e) T—This is a systemic vasculitis.

75. (a) F—Loop diuretics are the most powerful diuretics.
    (b) F—Calcium excretion increases due to a lower positive lumen potential.
    (c) T—This is the main site of action.
    (d) T—Diuretics act to increase fluid excretion.
    (e) F—This is seen in aldosterone antagonist diuretics.

76. (a) F—ACE inhibitors act to inhibit the conversion of angiotensin I (from renin) to angiotensin II.
    (b) T—ACE inhibitors improve the outcome in heart failure.
    (c) F—ACE inhibitors can cause developmental abnormalities or neonatal hypotension.
    (d) T—This is because aldosterone is inhibited.
    (e) T—ACE inhibitors are used in diabetic nephropathy.

77. (a) T—The ureters are always behind the peritoneum.
    (b) T—Pain caused by ureteric obstruction is referred to the skin of T11–L2, which innervates the scrotum (males) and labium majus (females).
    (c) F—Maximum bladder capacity is 500mL.
    (d) F—The bladder neck is fixed and immobile.
    (e) F—The prostate is partly glandular and partly muscular.

78. (a) T—High blood calcium means more calcium is seen in the urine.
    (b) T—Calcium can precipitate out in the urinary tract, predisposing calculi formation.
    (c) T—A concentrated urine predisposes stone formation.
    (d) F—Stones can be formed from urate, so a low urate does not predispose stone formation.
    (e) T—Spinach contains oxalate, which is found in calcium stones.

79. (a) T—These can be congenital.
    (b) F—This is a consequence, not a cause, of obstruction.
    (c) T—This is an extraluminal mass, which impinges on the urinary tract.
    (d) T—Calculi within the lumen obstruct the urinary tract.
    (e) T—The fetus acts as an extraluminal mass, which impinges on the urinary tract.

80. (a) T—Pain occurs as the urinary tract muscle contracts to expel the obstruction.
    (b) T—The renal pelvis dilates as urine flow through the tract is blocked.
    (c) T—Obstruction can impair renal function, impairing urine concentrating ability.
    (d) T—This is rare, suggesting complete urethral or bilateral ureteric obstruction.
    (e) F—Obstruction presents with overflow incontinence.

81. (a) T—This causes renal ischaemia due to hypervolaemic shock.
    (b) T—All aminoglycosides are nephrotoxic, so patients should be monitored carefully.
    (c) F—There is no association with ATN.
    (d) F—These cause membranous nephropathy.
    (e) T—This can occasionally cause renal impairment.

82. (a) T—Urine production falls because there are fewer functioning nephrons.
    (b) T—Prompt treatment is required.
    (c) F—ATN is life-threatening because of hyperkalaemia.
    (d) F—This predisposes to ATN.
    (e) F—ATN is an acute event, so is not associated with a change in kidney size.

83. (a) F—A low-protein diet helps alleviate uraemic syndrome.
    (b) T—This regulates plasma calcium and phosphate. High levels are associated with hypertension and renal stones.
    (c) T—Good blood pressure control delays the onset of ESRF.
    (d) T—This is due to a fall in erythropoietin production, resulting in a normochromic, normocytic anaemia.
    (e) T—Dialysis is required to supplement the functions of the failing kidneys.

84. (a) F—This causes metabolic alkalosis.
    (b) T—Diabetes is a cause of ketoacidosis.
    (c) T—There is failure to excrete acid.
    (d) T—This is because of excess intake of acid.
    (e) F—Aldosterone does not affect H^+/HCO_3^- metabolism.

85. (a) F—This increases potassium excretion, thereby causing hypokalaemia.
    (b) F—Alkalosis is a high pH with low H^+, usually accompanied by low K^+.
    (c) F—β-agonists are used to lower potassium (drives it into cells).
    (d) F—Insulin drives K^+ back into cells.
    (e) F—Osmolarity does not alter blood K^+ levels.

86. (a) T—The duodenum is an anterior relation.
    (b) F—The inferior vena cava lies immediately lateral to the right kidney.
    (c) F—It is lower due to the liver.
    (d) T—The psoas lies posteriorly to both kidneys.
    (e) T—The descending colon passes anteriorly.

87. (a) F—The incidence of BPH increases with age.
    (b) T—In comparison, prostate cancer is associated with tumours in the lateral lobes.
    (c) T—Surgery relieves the bladder outflow obstruction.
    (d) F—BPH is benign.
    (e) T—BPH acts as an obstruction, causing incomplete voiding which predisposes to UTI.

88. (a) T—This is more common than urinary tract malignancies.
    (b) T—RCC can be asymptomatic.
    (c) F—This is produced in the liver.
    (d) T—This is the most common tumour site.
    (e) T—This is associated with renal carcinoma, phaeochromocytoma and aneurysms.

89. (a) T—In children it is autosomal recessive.
    (b) F—It usually presents with haematuria, UTI, pain or abdominal mass.
    (c) T—Treatment is supportive.
    (d) T—There is a gradual deterioration in renal function.
    (e) T—Subarachnoid haemorrhage can occur.

90. (a) F—TCC is a malignant tumour.
    (b) T—This is a risk factor for TCC.
    (c) T—TCC is associated with schistosomiasis, which is common in Egypt.
    (d) F—Haematuria is usually painless.
    (e) T—This is the classic location for bladder TCC.

91. (a) F—This produces a continuous loss of urine without voluntary control.
    (b) F—This is associated with stress incontinence.
    (c) F—This causes overflow incontinence.
    (d) T—This causes neuronal dysfunction, affecting bladder function.
    (e) T—This reduces detrusor muscle stability.

92. (a) T—It does not involve detrusor muscle instability.
    (b) T—This is due to pelvic floor laxity following multiple childbirths or uterine prolapse.
    (c) T—There is poor sphincter function.
    (d) T—This can damage the external sphincter.
    (e) T—This increases intra-abdominal pressure.

93. (a) T—Plasma osmolality is tightly controlled between 285 and 295 mOsmol/kg H_2O.
    (b) F—They are located in the anterior hypothalamus.
    (c) T—Osmoreceptors monitor plasma osmolality in the internal carotid artery.
    (d) F—They regulate ADH release.
    (e) T—ADH reduces water loss in urine.

94. (a) T—Nicotine stimulates the osmoreceptors and therefore stimulates ADH release.
    (b) T—This is released when there is renal hypoperfusion.
    (c) F—Alcohol may inhibit ADH secretion.
    (d) F—This increases ADH effects, but does not increase its release.
    (e) F—β-blockers reduce renin release (renin stimulates ADH release).

95. (a) T—Tumours usually develop in one kidney.
    (b) T—These can exist in one kidney only.
    (c) T—Bacterial pyelonephritis may be unilaterral.
    (d) T—This can be bilateral.
    (e) F—This is characterized by small kidneys (bilateral).

96. (a) T—The left kidney can be confused with the spleen, the right kidney with the liver.
    (b) T—This distinguishes the kidney from the spleen or liver.
    (c) F—This is characteristic of the spleen.
    (d) T—This is because children have thinner abdominal walls.
    (e) F—Enlargement usually occurs gradually, and is painless.

97. (a) F—They can be found in normal urine.
    (b) F—The presence of any red cell casts is pathological.
    (c) T—This develops because of faulty glomerular filtration.
    (d) T—ATN results in tubular cell death and shedding into the tubular lumen.
    (e) F—This indicates the nephritic syndrome.

98. (a) T—It can be used to differentiate between tumours and cysts.
    (b) F—Ultrasound is used mainly to identify any obvious large anatomical abnormalities, and their nature.
    (c) F—Ultrasound identifies the pelvicalyceal system and the ureter only if dilated.
    (d) T—Ultrasound is the method of choice.
    (e) F—Ultrasound does not highlight fine detail, indicative of rejection.

99. (a) T—Biopsy can also be performed if the aetiology of renal dysfunction is unknown.
    (b) F—This is performed only if influential to management.
    (c) T—A needle probe is inserted into the kidney to extract a tissue sample.
    (d) T—Haematoma is a common complication of biopsy.
    (e) T—Biopsy is technically difficult.

100. (a) F—KUB specifies a complete view of the upper and lower urinary tract.
     (b) F—10% of stones are not visible on X-rays.
     (c) T—This is the investigation of choice.
     (d) T—MRI can also be used.
     (e) F—Contrast is injected into the renal artery.

1. (a) Regulation of water content, mineral composition and pH of the body by excreting each substance in an amount adequate to achieve total body balance and maintain normal concentration in the extracellular fluid.
    (b) Elimination of metabolic waste products from the blood and their excretion in urine (e.g. urea from protein metabolism, uric acid from nucleic acids, creatinine from muscle creatinine).
    (c) Removal of foreign chemicals from blood and excretion in urine (e.g. drugs, pesticides, food additives).
    (d) Secretion of hormones: erythropoietin to control erythrocyte production; renin to catalyse the conversion of angiotensin I from angiotensinogen and so control blood pressure and sodium balance; 1,25-dihydroxycholecalciferol (1,25(OH)$_2$D$_3$) to influence calcium metabolism.

2. The kidneys receive 20–25% of the total cardiac output (1.2 L/min). The blood enters the kidney via the right and left renal arteries. These branch to form about five interlobar arteries, which divide to form the arcuate arteries located at the junction between the cortex and medulla. The interlobular arteries are perpendicular to the arcuate arteries and pass through the cortex dividing up to form the afferent arterioles, which supply the glomerular capillaries. The efferent arterioles drain blood from the glomerular capillaries acting as portal vessels (i.e. carrying blood from one capillary network to another). In the outer two-thirds of the cortex the efferent arterioles form a network of peritubular capillaries that supply all the cortical parts of the nephron. In the inner third of the cortex the capillaries go on to follow a hairpin course adjacent to the loops of Henle and the collecting ducts down into the medulla. These vessels are known as the vasa recta. The vasa recta and the peritubular capillaries drain into the left and right renal veins and then into the inferior vena cava. Figure 2.7 shows the microcirculation of the kidney.

3. There are three consecutive systems that form the adult urinary tract—pronephros, mesonephros and metanephros.
    (a) The pronephros develops in the cervical region of the embryo and is rudimentary.
    (b) The mesonephros has characteristic excretory units with their own collecting ducts, called the mesonephric duct or the Wolffian duct. It develops in the thoracic and lumbar regions as the pronephros regresses. It can function for a short time.
    (c) The metanephros (permanent kidney) develops in the pelvic region at about 5 weeks. It forms excretory units (nephrons) from the metanephric

mesoderm and the collecting system is formed from the ureteric bud, which is an outgrowth of the mesonephric duct. The metanephric tissue forms a cap over the ureteric bud and, on growth and dilatation of the bud, it forms the renal pelvis, ureters and the collecting ducts. The connection between the collecting system and the nephrons is essential for the normal development of the urinary tract. Any failure in the process will cause unilateral or bilateral renal agenesis or cystic disease (see Chapter 4). If the ureteric bud divides too early the result is bifid kidneys (duplex ureters), occasionally with ectopic ureters.

4. Answers (refer to Chapters 4 and 5 for a detailed explanation) should include two of the following:
    (a) Double and bifid ureters.
    (b) Uteropelvic obstruction.
    (c) Ureteral or bladder diverticula.
    (d) Hydroureters.
    (e) Bladder extrophy.
    (f) Urethral valves.
    (g) Horseshoe kidney.
    (h) Pelvic kidney.

5. The composition of the ultrafiltrate of plasma is dependent upon the three layers of the filtration barrier. The characteristics and functions of these three layers listed below need to be discussed (refer to Figure 2.9):
    (a) The endothelial cells of the capillary.
    (b) The basement membrane.
    (c) The epithelial cells of Bowman's capsule.

6. Answer to include with examples:
    (a) Diffusion.
    (b) Facilitated diffusion.
    (c) Primary active transport.
    (d) Secondary active transport.

7. Answer (see Chapter 3) to include the use of:
    (a) Creatinine.
    (b) Inulin.
    (c) p-aminohippuric acid (PAH).
    (d) Inert gas washout technique.
    (e) Isotope uptake technique.
    (f) ^{31}Cr EDTA.

8. (a) 10th week gestation—filtration of fluid and urine production.
    (b) Newborn RBF is 5% of cardiac output—increases progressively during the first year.
    (c) Postpartum GFR is 25 mL/min/1.73 m^2 body surface area.
    (d) One month old—progressive increase in GFR.
    (e) By one year GFR is adult value—125 mL/min.

187

(f) Adult RBF is 20% of cardiac output.
(g) Old age—GFR decreases progressively. Draw the graph (Fig. 3.6) to help explain.

9. Plasma glucose normal range is 2.5–5.5mmol. About 0.2–0.5mmol of glucose is filtered every minute if the plasma concentration is normal. Any increase in the plasma glucose concentration results in a proportional increase in the amount of glucose filtered. Virtually all the filtered glucose is reabsorbed in the proximal tubule unless the filtered glucose exceeds the resorptive capacity of the cells.

(a) Glucose is transported into the proximal tubular cells against its concentration gradient by active transport (a symport). Glucose reabsorption is driven by energy released from the transport of sodium down its electrochemical gradient as the Na^+/K^+ ATPase pump on the basolateral membrane maintains a low sodium concentration and negative potential within the cell. Figure 2.22 shows glucose transport in cells of the pars convoluta. The transport ratio is 1:1 sodium: glucose in the pars convoluta and 2:1 sodium: glucose in the pars recta.

(b) All the nephrons have different thresholds for glucose reabsorption (nephron heterogeneity). T_m is the maximum tubular resorptive capacity for a solute (i.e. the point of saturation for the carriers) and this value can be calculated for glucose. There is a limited number of Na^+/glucose carrier molecules and so glucose reabsorption is T_m limited. Figure 2.23 shows the relationship between glucose reabsorption and excretion depending upon the plasma concentration. The graph shows that the lowest renal threshold of glucose is at a plasma glucose of 10mmol/L. At this level, filtered glucose will begin to be excreted in the urine (glycosuria). As plasma glucose concentration increases further (as can occur in uncontrolled diabetes mellitus) even the nephrons with highest resorptive capacity will allow glucose excretion and urinary glucose increases in parallel with plasma glucose. The T_m is reached at a plasma glucose concentration of 20mmol/L.

(c) In pregnancy the renal threshold for glucose is temporarily decreased and glucose can appear in the urine even when blood glucose is less than 10mmol/L (renal glycosuria).

10. Plasma concentration of bicarbonate is 20–30mmol/L. Bicarbonate ions (HCO_3^-) are vital in the maintenance of acid–base balance within the body. The kidney plays an important part in the regulation of pH by controlling the plasma HCO_3^- concentration; 90% of the filtered HCO_3^- is reabsorbed into the proximal tubule and the remaining 10% is taken up in the distal tubule and collecting ducts. The reabsorption of HCO_3^- is also coupled to Na^+ transport. Figure 2.24 illustrates the reabsorption of HCO_3^- in the proximal tubule cells. The mechanism of HCO_3^- reabsorption is as follows: Na^+ reabsorption on the apical membrane drives H^+ secretion into the tubular cells and these combine with HCO_3^- to form carbonic acid (H_2CO_3).

The presence of carbonic anhydrase on the brush border of the cells catalyses the dissociation of H_2CO_3 into H_2O and CO_2 within the tubular lumen. Both H_2O and CO_2 diffuse freely into the cell where they are recombined to form H_2CO_3, catalysed by intracellular carbonic anhydrase. HCO_3^- and Na^+ are transported out of the cell across the basolateral membrane. H^+ is secreted out of the cell into the tubular lumen and recycled to allow continuation of this cycle.

11. See Figure 2.6.

12. Nodular and diffuse glomerulosclerosis, arteriolar lesions, and exudative lesions such as the fibrin cap are all renal manifestations of diabetes mellitus.

(a) On electron microscopy there is an increase in the thickness of the glomerular basement membrane and an increase in mesangial matrix with two morphological patterns: (1) nodular glomerulosclerosis (Kimmelstiel–Wilson nodules)—nodular accumulations of mesangial matrix material; and (2) diffuse glomerulosclerosis—diffusely increased areas of mesangial matrix.

(b) The onset of diabetic nephropathy is clinically manifest by the development of microalbuminuria followed by overt proteinuria, which can reach the nephrotic range. There is then a progressive fall in GFR, which is commonly associated with hypertension. Diabetic nephropathy is usually associated with diabetic complications in other organs (especially retinopathy). Diabetes mellitus has usually been present for approximately 20 years before the development of end-stage renal failure. The most common cause of needing dialysis in developed countries is chronic renal failure due to diabetes mellitus.

(c) Pyelonephritis is a common complication in patients with diabetes mellitus and can cause renal papillary necrosis.

13. (a) ACE inhibitors block ACE, which hydrolyses angiotensin I to angiotensin II. Angiotensin I is inactive and is converted in the lung to angiotensin II; this in turn is converted to angiotensin III in the adrenal gland. Angiotensin II is a very potent vasoconstrictor and aids sodium reabsorption in the tubule. The stimulus for activation of the renin–angiotensin–aldosterone system is reduced renal arteriolar pressure, sympathetic stimulation and a reduction in the delivery of Na^+ concentration to the distal tubule.

(b) Any condition resulting in high circulating levels of renin will result in angiotensin-mediated high vascular resistance contributing to hypertension. ACE inhibitors (e.g. captopril, enalapril) inhibit the enzyme peptidyl dipeptidase, which converts angiotensin I to II and therefore lowers blood pressure by decreasing peripheral vascular resistance (TPR). ACE inhibitors can also decrease blood pressure by inhibiting the local (tissue) renin–angiotensin system. ACE inhibitors have been shown to decrease proteinuria and delay the progress of renal disease in people with diabetes

mellitus. They are also increasingly being used in the treatment of congestive cardiac failure.
(c) Figure 4.16 shows the effects of ACE inhibitors.

14. (a) In 2–5% of patients with hypertension, the hypertension is secondary to RAS in one or both renal arteries. The stenoses might be due to fibromuscular dysplasia or atheromatous plaques (70%) within the renal artery wall. The result is excessive renin secretion by the affected kidney because there is renal hypoperfusion and this is interpreted as a fall in body fluid volume. There is also a small degree of renal ischaemia. Treatment to dilate the stenosis (angioplasty), or corrective surgery, can aid blood pressure control and preserve renal function. If the blood pressure is left uncontrolled the contralateral kidney might become damaged by hypertension.
(b) People with RAS rely on constriction of the efferent renal arteriole to maintain pressures for glomerular filtration on the affected side. Angiotensin II is the main agent responsible for constriction of these vessels. On ACE inhibitor administration, a decrease in angiotensin II will dramatically decrease glomerular capillary pressure within the kidney resulting in acute renal failure.

15. (a) In situ immune-complex deposition. Immune complexes are formed within the kidney. The antibodies react with intrinsic or planted antigens within the glomerulus. Antiglomerular basement membrane (GBM) disease is an example involving intrinsic antigen. Antibodies are formed against an antigen in the GBM. The complex elicits the complement cascade, leading to severe damage to the glomerulus and rapidly progressing renal failure. The anti-GBM antibodies also attack the basement membrane of the alveoli in the lungs. The association of anti-GBM antibodies, glomerulonephritis (GN) and pulmonary haemorrhage is known as Goodpasture's syndrome. Planted antigens are antigens planted within the glomerulus and not of renal origin. They can be:
   (i) Exogenous: for example, bacteria such as group A β-haemolytic streptococcus. This results in post-streptococcal GN. Other antigens include bacterial products (endostreptosin), aggregated IgG, viruses, parasites and drugs.
   (ii) Endogenous: for example, nucleic acid—antibodies react with host DNA as seen in systemic lupus erythematosus (SLE).
(b) Circulating immune complex nephritis. Here, immune complexes are not formed within the kidney. They are formed elsewhere and get trapped within the glomerulus from the renal circulation. When trapped in the glomerulus, the immune complex causes an inflammatory reaction, resulting in damage to the glomerulus. On immunofluorescence microscopy, granular deposits are seen along the basement membrane and/or in the mesangium. Once again the antigen can be:

   (i) Exogenous: for example, bacteria (group A streptococci, *Treponema pallidum*), surface antigen of hepatitis B, hepatitis C virus antigen, tumour antigens, viruses.
   (ii) Endogenous: DNA in SLE.
(c) Cytotoxic antibodies. Antibodies to glomerular cell antigens are formed and cause damage without any deposits. For example, antibodies fixing to mesangial cells and causing complement-mediated mesangiolysis and mesangial cell proliferation. Experimental examples of this are known in rats but it is not clear that this occurs in man.
(d) Cell-mediated immunity. Sensitized T cells from cell-mediated immune reactions can cause glomerular injury. This form of damage is important in progressive GN. It is thought that macrophages and T lymphocytes are present and mediate damage in the glomerulus in such cases.
(e) Activation of the alternative complement pathway. Bacterial polysaccharides, endotoxins and IgA aggregates can activate the alternative complement pathway and give rise to components that then deposit in the glomeruli causing damage. This mechanism is seen in membranoproliferative GN.

16. The complications of prolonged obstruction of urine flow are associated with compensatory hypertrophy of the bladder wall as a result of high pressure that develops within the bladder (Fig. 5.8) and are as follows:
(a) Bands of thickened smooth muscle fibre cause trabeculation of the bladder wall.
(b) Diverticula formation on the external surface of the bladder.
(c) Bladder dilation once the muscle becomes hypotonic.
(d) Hydroureter formation resulting in reflux of urine up to the renal pelvis.
(e) Bilateral hydronephrosis.
(f) Kidney infection, stones and renal failure.

17. (a) The bruits are a sign of vascular disease; they develop as a result of atheromatous narrowing in the blood vessels. The abdominal bruits suggest renal artery stenosis (RAS), whereas the carotid bruit is the most likely origin for an embolus, which could have caused the stroke.
(b) The diagnosis is hypertension and impaired renal function secondary to RAS. The patient also has hypercholesterolaemia, which predisposes to atherosclerosis and RAS.
(c) Renal angiography is the investigation of choice.
(d) Patients with RAS have high circulating levels of angiotensin II, which acts to constrict efferent arterioles and maintain GFR. ACE inhibitors prevent this protective mechanism and therefore cause an acute fall in GFR.
(e) The patient does not require dialysis because renal function has not deteriorated to such an extent that supplementary renal therapy is required to maintain renal function.
(f) Management includes blood pressure control, dietary restriction of cholesterol, investigation of

RAS and carotid artery stenosis, and regular monitoring of renal function. Cholesterol levels should also be monitored.

18. (a) A digital rectal examination must be performed. This will confirm any prostatic enlargement, and differentiate between benign prostatic hypertrophy (BPH—feels smooth) and prostatic carcinoma (hard and irregular).
   (b) As stated above, the two most likely diagnoses in a male patient above the age of 40 are BPH and prostate cancer.
   (c) Prostatic cancer is associated with a rise in PSA (prostate-specific antigen). However, it should be noted that a normal PSA does not exclude prostate carcinoma.

19. (a) The most likely diagnosis is nephrotic syndrome, of which the most common cause in children would be minimal change glomerulonephritis. It is more common in Asians, and in males.
   (b) Useful investigations include urine dipstick (showing gross proteinuria and blood albumin <25 g/L), renal function tests (i.e. urea, creatinine, etc.), urine microscopy and, hepatitis B antigen.
   (c) Treatment involves diuretics to relieve the oedema, salt and fluid restriction, oral steroids (prednisolone) and, in the acute phase, penicillin prophylaxis.

20. (a) The most likely explanation for this presentation is a bladder calculus. As the bladder empties, the bladder wall contracts, forcing the stone against the bladder wall. This irritates the bladder lining, causing pain and bleeding.
   (b) The patient also has pain in his penis since this receives its sensory supply from the pudendal nerve (S1, 2, 3) and the ilioinguinal nerve (L1 and 2). The bladder is also innervated by these segments, so pain is referred to the penis. Upon lying down, the bladder stone rolls back, no longer irritating the trigone membrane. Consequently, the pain is alleviated.
   (c) The investigation of choice to confirm the presence of stones is an ultrasound. Alternatively, a KUB radiograph can be ordered.

Index

Page numbers in *italics* refer to figures and tables